Unipolar
depression

Unipolar depression
A lifespan perspective

Edited by
Ian M. Goodyer

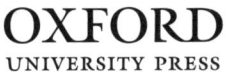

OXFORD
UNIVERSITY PRESS

OXFORD

UNIVERSITY PRESS

Great Clarendon Street, Oxford OX2 6DP

Oxford University Press is a department of the University of Oxford.
It furthers the University's objective of excellence in research, scholarship,
and education by publishing worldwide in

Oxford New York

Auckland Bangkok Buenos Aires Cape Town Chennai
Dar es Salaam Delhi Hong Kong Istanbul Karachi Kolkata
Kuala Lumpur Madrid Melbourne Mexico City Mumbai Nairobi
São Paulo Shanghai Taipei Tokyo Toronto

Oxford is a registered trade mark of Oxford University Press in the UK
and in certain other countries

Published in the United States
by Oxford University Press Inc., New York

© Oxford University Press 2003

The moral rights of the author have been asserted

Database right Oxford University Press (maker)

First published 2003

A Catalogue record for this title is available from the British Library

Library of Congress Cataloging in Publication Data
(Data available)

ISBN 0-19-851095-0

1 3 5 7 9 10 8 6 4 2

Typeset in Minion
by Newgen Imaging Systems (P) Ltd., Chennai, India
Printed in Great Britain on
acid-free paper by
Biddles Ltd, Guildford and King's Lynn

Preface

Unipolar major depression is one of the most serious mental health disorders whose adverse outcomes include chronic mental and physical ill health, social difficulties, and successful suicide. The disorder occurs across the lifespan but the nature characteristics and outcomes of the condition may vary with age. It is unclear if children, adolescents, adults, and the elderly who present with a depressive illness are necessarily suffering from the same disorder with common aetiologies or will respond to the same treatments. Whilst much has been learnt about the causes and outcomes of unipolar depression a lifespan approach to the syndrome has yet to be systematically undertaken. The extent to which genetic and environmental factors and processes contribute to onset may be influenced by the developmental components of human growth and ageing. The social context within which depressions occur are not the same at different points in development but there are clearly negative consequences of negative experience that relate to the onset of a depressive episode from childhood through to late life. Similarly cortisol hypersecretion and abnormalities of serotonin function have been reported in depressed cases at most ages but their precise meaning across the lifespan is unclear. Finally the relative effects of psychological and pharmacological treatments are different for unipolar depressions at different ages pre-pubertal children being notably non-responsive to anti-depressants compared with other age groups and the elderly perhaps more responsive to cognitive therapies than has often been supposed.

This volume brings together a group of clinical scientists who have investigated unipolar depression at different stages in the lifespan to determine the continuities and discontinuities in the nature, characteristics and outcome of this syndrome at different ages and stages of development. It is hoped that by having the opportunity to compare and contrast what we know about unipolar major depressions at different timepoints the reader will gain new insights into the complex interplay between nature and nurture over the lifespan.

I.G.
Cambridge 2002

Contents

Contributors

Boris Birmaher
Associate Professor of Psychiatry,
University of Pittsburgh Medical Center,
Western Psychiatric Institute and Clinic,
3811 O' Hara St.,
Pittsburgh, PA, 15213, USA
Email: birmaherb@msx.upmc.edu

Peter Cooper
Professor of Psychopathology,
Winnicott Research Unit,
School of Psychology,
University of Reading,
Whiteknights,
Reading, RG6 6AL, UK
Email: p.j.cooper@rdg.ac.uk

Ian M. Goodyer
Professor of Child and Adolescent
Psychiatry, Developmental Psychiatry
Section, Department of Psychiatry,
University of Cambridge,
Douglas House, 18b Trumpington
Road, Cambridge, CB2 2AH, UK,
Email: igl04@cus.cam.ac.uk

Richard Harrington
Professor of Child and Adolescent
Psychiatry, University Department of
Child and Adolescent Psychiatry,
Royal Manchester Children's Hospital,
Pendlebury, Manchester, M27 4HA,
UK

N. Kennedy
Clinical Lecturer in Psychiatry,
Box 189, Addenbrooke's Hospital,
Cambridge, CB2 2QQ, UK

Dr. Peter M. Lewinsohn
Director, Oregon Research Institute,
1715 Franklin Blvd., Eugene, Oregon
97403-1983, USA
Email: pete@ori.org

Lynne Murray
Professor of Developmental
Psychopathology,
Winnicot Research Unit,
School of Psychology,
University of Reading, Whiteknights,
Reading, RG6 6AL, UK
Email: lynne.murray@rdg.ac.uk

John O'Brien
Professor of Old Age Psychiatry,
Wolfson Research Centre, Institute for
Ageing and Health, Newcastle General
Hospital, Westgate Road,
Newcastle upon Tyne NE4 6BE, UK
E-mail: j.t.o'brien@net.ac.uk

E.S. Paykel
Emeritus Professor of Psychiatry,
Department of Psychiatry,
University of Cambridge,
Douglas House,
18e Trumpington Road,
Cambridge, CB2 2AH, UK

John Samuel Rozel
Resident in General and Child and
Adolescent Psychiatry, University of
Pittsburgh Medical Center, Western
Psychiatric Institute and Clinic,
3811 O' Hara St.,
Pittsburgh, PA, 15213, USA
Email: rozeljs@msx.upmc.edu

John R. Seeley
Oregon Research Institute, 1715
Franklin Blvd., Eugene, Oregon
97403-1983, USA

Alan Thomas
Senior Lecturer in Old Age Psychiatry,
Wolfson Research Centre, Institute for
Ageing and Health, Newcastle General
Hospital, Westgate Road,
Newcastle upon Tyne NE4 6BE, UK
Email: a.j.thomas@ncl.ac.uk

Chapter 1

Characteristics of unipolar depressions

Ian M. Goodyer

Unipolar depressive syndromes constitute a serious group of mental disorders with considerable risk for recurrence and psychosocial impairment throughout the lifespan. Using the American Psychiatric Association DSM clinical criteria (American Psychiatric Association, 1994) successfully identifies the same clinical syndromes in school age children, adolescents, and adults. The majority of psychiatric studies have focussed on two disorders, major depression and dysthymia although there is an emerging literature on other affective syndromes, including depressive adjustment reaction, minor depressions, and more recently early onset bi-polar disorder.

Clinical constituents of depression

All affective conditions, including the depressive component of bi-polar disorder, share a core set of signs and symptoms that involve undesirable alterations of mood and feelings, thoughts, social behaviours, and physical functions. An essential feature is that of a change in mood from pleasant (euphoric) to unpleasant (dysphoric), even painful. This mood shift is experienced as relatively pervasive, persisting over time and place and sufficiently severe to interrupt every day functioning. This negative mood state is accompanied by other sets of other features in varying combinations including negative and distorted cognitions about the self, impaired concentration and attention, and an adverse alteration in a range of physical characteristics, eating, sleeping, energy, and activity. Symptoms are generally elicited at interview through direct questioning of the patient (and parents in the case of children and adolescents), occasionally obtaining information from other relatives, teachers or close friends. Signs are concurrent observations made by the interviewer about the respondents general appearance and may include changes in facial expression, increases or decreases in physical activity, general care in dressing and personal hygiene, diminished speed and fluency of speech. Interviewers are also expected to make a judgement about the subject's general awareness of their mental condition, recent and current behaviour, and general personal care. This evaluation of the degree of insight a subject has into their well-being may have considerable implications for clinical management. For example, the ability of the patient to participate in voluntary treatment may be determined by the interviewers evaluation of this latter feature. The extent to the wider social and family environment, are involved in clinical care and subsequent management (such as home support) may also be determined by the interviewers judgement of insight and other person specific characteristics such as motivation for treatment.

Detecting depressive signs and symptoms

The reliability and validity of diagnostic assessments have been the subject of much investigation in University and research settings using instruments developed for research inquiries in both clinical and community populations at all ages. By contrast little is known of the utility and efficacy of diagnostic procedures in routine clinical practise used throughout the world, or the processes through which diagnoses are arrived at in different settings, such as private practise, health care clinics, multidisciplinary teams or primary care. As a result the sensitivity and specificity for the detection of mental disorders in health care settings by different professional groups is not known. Furthermore the same language may be used to convey quite different things about the patient's current well-being. For example, the word depression may be used to describe a particular mood state only, a psychological dynamic or causal process, a syndrome of signs and symptoms, a categorical illness state, or even a disease with known pathophysiological correlates or established aetiological mechanisms.

The focus of most research into affective disorders has been on the detection of syndromes obtained from interview procedures, often delivered by intensively trained research staff (Lewinsohn *et al.*, 1994; Kendler and Roy, 1995). In large scale epidemiological studies quantitative symptom counts of current low mood, negative thoughts and physical changes obtained from self-report or parent questionnaires have been used as additional proxies for syndromes to improve the power of the investigation (Silberg *et al.*, 1999). In clinical studies where samples sizes of 'real' cases are large enough (generally between 80 and 200) multivariate statistics have been applied to obtain distinctive factors or clusters of signs and symptoms as a test of the construct validity of depressive syndromes. For example in children and adolescents there appear to be differences in the form of depressive disorders with pre-pubertal children subjects showing greater numbers of anxious and physical symptoms than post-pubertal adolescents (Ryan *et al.*, 1987; Kolvin *et al.*, 1991). Distinctions in form have also been noted between unipolar presentations in mid life and the elderly with apathy and less anxiety being more prominent in older cases (see Chapters 6 and 7, this volume for a full discussion of these clinical differences in adult life). Community and clinical studies in younger populations have also paid considerable attention to the signs and symptoms reflecting other disorders accompanying the presence of major unipolar depression. The inclusion of co-morbid syndromes has been used at some points in the life span as adjunctive methods for categorizing clinical subtypes of depression. Examples for child and adolescent research include double depression (dysthymia and subsequent major depression) (Kovacs, 1997), depressive conduct disorder (Harrington *et al.*, 1991) and depressive obsessional disorder (Goodyer *et al.*, 1997). For presenting depressive disorders in young people comorbid syndromes are the rule rather than the exception but their validity as a clinical marker of aetiological differences within this group of conditions remains unclear (Angold *et al.*, 1999).

Depressive syndromes

The early work in adult populations was successful in delineating the characteristics of somatic (high levels of physical symptoms weight loss, insomnia, early morning waking, diurnal variation of mood, persistent feelings of guilt, hopelessness, and psychomotor retardation or agitation), from psychological depressions (anxious mood, initial insomnia, self-pity rather than self-blame, complaints of anorexia rather than weight loss). A series of criteria for the classification of depression was subsequently proposed by Feighner and colleagues at Saint Louis (Feighner *et al.*, 1972). Phenomenological psychopathology remained the core construct guiding these criteria with no dependency on putative causation. These suggestions formed the basis for subsequent refinements that led to Research Diagnostic Criteria for the diagnosis of depression (Spitzer *et al.*, 1978). For these purposes a diagnostic category had to be supported by two sets of mutually exclusive descriptive criteria: those that specify characteristics that lead towards making a diagnosis (inclusion criteria) and those that lead away from making the diagnosis (exclusion criteria). These principles form the basis of the current American Psychiatric Association's classification in the Diagnostic and Statistical Manual (American Psychiatric Association, 1994) and the International Classification of Diseases sponsored by the World Health Organization (WHO, 1994). The adoption of these systems has led to a method of classification that has satisfactory reliability between professional raters for signs, symptoms and course of depressive disorder. The system has proven highly successful in generating a common language for the diagnosis of depressive disorders that make findings comparable between investigations despite marked differences in the nature of the populations studied. This categorical approach to classification of depression is not without its detractors however. For example, it is widely recognized that meeting inclusion criteria still allows for considerable variation in clinical presentation, including high levels of non-depressive symptoms, giving rise to marked individual differences in the descriptive psychopathology of depressions. With the main research emphasis on the quantity of depressive symptoms as predictors of subsequent onset of depression, little attention has been paid as yet to the relative importance of different types of symptoms or their salience to the subject, for evolving a depressive disorder. Subjects in the community may (if asked) complain of a range of symptoms that fall below inclusion threshold for a diagnosis (too few or insufficient duration) but are of sufficient severity to cause personal impairment.

Major unipolar depression

According to DSM IV (American Psychiatric Association, 1994) the diagnosis of major depressive disorder (MDD) requires establishing first the mandatory presence of lowered mood (dysphoria) together with four of eight other possible non-mandatory symptoms from the two broad domains of disordered cognitions and physical changes. These are shown in Table 1.1.

It is essential that the five symptoms occur concurrently with each other over a minimum two week period. In children and adolescents, but not in adults, the entry criteria of lowered mood can be irritability. Young people will often identify their own negative feelings with mood valent words such as gloomy, grumpy or down, and these should be used in interviews where there is uncertainty about the salience of the word depressed, such as with the pre-pubertal child. In adults, and the elderly patient in particular, it may be important to inquire about mood state in those who appear apathetic or disinterested in the assessment procedure. It is important to establish that these symptoms are not accounted for by the direct effects of substance misuse or a general medical condition, particularly one that

Table 1.1 Symptoms of major depression in childhood and adolescence[1]

Mood[2]	Cognitive	Physical
Dysphoria or Irritability in children	Anhedonia Feelings of worthlessness	Weight change (includes a failure to make expected weight gains)
	Inappropriate guilt Diminished ability to think or concentrate	Fatigue or loss of energy Psychomotor agitation or retardation
	Recurrent thoughts of death or suicidal ideation	

Notes:
[1] The diagnosis can only be made when five or more symptoms are present over a two week period
[2] Dysphoric mood must be present

involves known brain changes as this reduces the likelihood of reliable and valid mental state assessments. In addition the symptoms should not be accounted for by recent bereavement. (*nb* these caveats are not implying that such subjects cannot be subsequently clinically depressed as a consequence of these experiences, rather that symptoms essential to the diagnosis may be acute or transient and therefore increase the liability of a false positive diagnosis at the time of presentation).

There are no requirements for a particular pattern of cognitions and/or physical symptoms. Despite the inference from many studies across the lifespan that physical symptoms reflect a more sustained, severe or even 'biological' syndrome, there is no hierarchy or weighting in favour of these features in the DSM classification system (*nb* but see ICD 10 somatic depression sub type which has been accorded special status because of the long standing clinical belief that endogenous depression is a severe and potentially distinctive disorder (WHO, 1994), see also the discussions in Chapter 6 concerning clinical presentation, treatment response, and outcome in mid life depressions). Equally no distinction is made regarding the duration of these disorders which, providing they have been present for at least two weeks, may vary in length for any period of time, even years. They may also differ in their severity or personal psychosocial impairment from mild, indicating only a modest deviation from normal behavioural functioning, to unable to care for oneself and requiring 24 h intensive psychiatric care.

Dysthymia

Dysthymia has been described as a chronic mood disturbance present for 2 years (one in childhood or adolescence) or more and characterized by: long standing gloom and dysphoria, brooding about feeling unloved, and affect dysregulation. The dominant negative cognition is self-deprecation or negative self-esteem. In young people there are high rates of irritability and anger in everyday circumstances, that is, occurring as a hyperemotional response to social hassles in the everyday environment (Kovacs, 1994). According to DSM IV dysthymia is a chronic depressive condition. In addition to depressed mood the subject must have two out of a further six symptoms from the list shown in table one except that feelings of guilt and suicidal behaviour are not included as they are for major depression. The implication is that the latter two symptoms are not found in dysthymic disorders and if present suggest that the patient is likely to be suffering from major depression.

In children dysthymia is distinguished by the virtual absence and significantly lower prevalence of anhedonia, social withdrawal, anorexia, and insomnia; and comparatively lower levels of guilt, morbid preoccupation, and impaired concentration (Kovacs, 1994).

It is important to establish that the patient does not fulfil criteria for current major depression. If major depression has preceded the onset of dysthymia then there must have been full remission of all depressive symptoms for at least two months before the development of dysthymia. By contrast episodes of major depression can be superimposed on dysthymia disorder in which circumstances both diagnoses can be given.

Sub-threshold and minor depressions

Aware of the limitations of coverage in the classification of mental disorders both DSM and ICD systems include criteria for a 'not otherwise specified' category, for those cases not meeting full criteria for a specified syndrome. Interestingly despite this important caveat there have been continual calls for the addition of new 'disorders'. During the DSM process over 150 different new disorders were proposed, with varying levels of evidence supporting their addition to the classification (Pincus et al., 1999). A recent review and synthesis of studies on minor depression and other 'brand names' demonstrated that a myriad of names and definitions for sub-threshold depression have been used in the literature with varying duration, symptom thresholds, and exclusions. Of particular importance was the observation that to date little has been done to bridge the difference between clinical and primary care perceptions of what constitutes a mental disorder. There is little doubt that primary care physicians see individuals of all ages with distressing and dysfunctional mental states that are not well articulated in the psychiatric nosology and are often not a major consideration to mental health specialists (Pincus *et al.*, 1999). The natural history of these sub-threshold conditions remains a matter for further research ideally in longitudinal designs such that the temporal relationship between impairments and clinical status can be examined as an evolving rather than static process. What little has been done to date suggests that, from the public health perspective it would be currently be unwise to ignore sub-threshold depressions (and indeed other sub-clinical syndromes) if they present with personal impairment (Costello *et al.*, 1999).

Risk for major depressions

Whilst syndromal classification appears to assist in categorizing syndromes of varying nature and severity there is the danger that this reflects no more than a short hand convenience obfuscating the underlying validity of more complex biological processes indexed at the clinical level by a continuity in depressive symptoms and personal impairments. The 'clinical' detection of these being no more than a function of the values of the prevailing nosological system of our times than scientific proof (Kendler and Gardner, 1998). Thus defining and refining the phenotypes of unipolar depressions and relating these to neurobiological systems is essential if we are to determine the origins of these disorders and distinguish those with an evolving negative trajectory from those with more benign sporadic effects. This is a crucial task of the next two decades as it is increasingly apparent that affective disorders are aetiologically as well as clinically heterogeneous involving both genetic and environmental processes (Kendler *et al.*, 1996; Kendler and Karkowski-Shuman, 1997). One research strategy into the origins of unipolar depressions has focussed on delineating individuals who are at risk in an effort to characterise the environmental and genetic components that contribute to the onset of illness. It is apparent from disparate lines of inquiry that no single risk factor can explain all forms of affective disorder. Increasingly complex patterns of putative causal agents have been proposed as researchers explore the multifaceted nature of pathways into and out of, depressive disorders. A major task for the foreseeable future is to determine not only the character of these risk factors but also how they operate to bring about depression.

The nature of risk

Risk can be defined as the degree to which the likelihood of a given outcome will occur following exposure to a defined agent. The relative importance of exposure is estimated by the probability of the outcome occurring in a given population compared with the level of occurrence in a non-exposed population. Risks are suspected causes and outcomes are undesirable. The magnitude of the risk is expressed as the odds ratio, that is, the degree to which the likelihood of outcome is increased as a consequence of exposure to the agent. A critical issue in risk evaluation is the importance of defining and characterizing the risk factor. Risks for psychopathology occur from a variety of sources both within and external to the subject. They may be defined at the level of the individual, family, or the community at large. For example, individuals may be born with genes that render them susceptible to psychiatric illness, acquire lesions such as head injury, that alter their capacity for learning or be exposed to negative environments, such as maltreatment, that diminish emotional and cognitive development. Familial environmental risks might include a neglectful or hostile parenting environment, or one that is inadequate (such as in failure to ensure food and shelter) without being emotionally negative. In addition neighbourhood risks may occur which may be physical such as poor housing or functionally difficult, such as living in violent or dangerous societies.

Invariably risks of these types are not independent of each other and determining their degree of association prior to the occurrence of the undesirable outcome is an important process in order to prevent the wrong interpretation of the putative effects of a single or particular grouping of risks.

The general approach to determining the importance of a set of risk characteristics is probabilistic. This involves comparing two populations, one exposed the other not, and determining a meaningful level above chance that outcome occurs in association with exposure. Demonstrating a statistical association between the putative agent and undesirable outcome is of itself insufficient. The size of this association provides an important indication of the likelihood of an effect. This has been termed the potency of a risk factor and is the maximal discrepancy achievable between exposed and unexposed groups (often referred to as high and low risk indicating exposed and not exposed). Many quantitative statistics are used to denote the size of the effect (potency) including odds ratio, risk ratio, relative, and attributable risk, as well as methods for their point and confidence interval estimation. In practice it is difficult to find two risk factors that are truly independent of each other. This often means that one is evaluating putative risk factors each likely to carry a moderate effect even in the best designed studies using the most sensitive of measures. Statistical procedures must be able to cope with a risk profile that is more often than not going to determine the relative contribution of two or more risk factors in the onset of a given disorder.

A statistical association with a high quantified level of effect, expressed as more than a threefold increase in the risk of a psychiatric disorder in the presence of two or more negative life events, or more than 50 per cent of the onsets of a symptom or syndrome attributable to the measured risk, is a necessary first step but insufficient of itself to interpret with confidence a causal association through exposure between risk and outcome. Risk factors must precede and be independent from the outcome variable of interest. For example, high scores on a self-report behaviour scale often precede the onset or emergence of clinically significant disorder with the latter invariably being detected because of an increase in symptoms, greater symptom severity and personal and or social impairment. The preceding self-report scores cannot denote a pure risk factor as they may also contain features of the disorder itself, albeit in a low level or non-impairing form. By contrast adverse social circumstances, temperamental style, physical and psychosexual growth represent features that are independent of mental states and may be viewed as potential candidate risk markers for different forms of emotional and behavioural difficulty or disorder.

Depressive disorders are in the main episodic in nature with first episodes occurring at any point over the lifespan but only some such episodes leading to a recurrent or chronic disorder. Prior and during episodes changes in physical and psychological characteristics are prominent and interplay closely with alterations in social experience. The risk profile most associated with onset of these conditions is likely to be drawn from more than one level of this complex biology. For example, severe personal disappointments *and* morning cortisol hypersecretion measured in the year before onset of illness are both significantly associated with the onset of first episode major depression in adolescents and adult women suggesting different levels of relatively proximal physiological and social risk additively contribute to these forms of affective psychopathology (Goodyer *et al.*, 2000*a,b*; Harris *et al.*, 2000). The candidate risks for affective disorders are not however confined to these domains alone as being at least tanner stage three with high testosterone and/or oestradiol levels are also associated with a marked increase in a range of depressive conditions in female adolescents (Angold *et al.*, 1999). In other words the population specificity of candidate risks may involve considerably more processing levels than the social environment. Whether differentiated risk patterns involving social, psychological and physiological components (and no doubt cellular and molecular genetic components) are sufficient to delineate clear cut forms of affective psychopathology is not yet clear. The recent evidence from prospective studies of adolescents of both sexes and women at high risk for major depression would suggest however that this more vertical and combined approach to risk measurement is more likely to capture the majority of subsequent cases than a single level and measure (e.g. family history of depression) of putative risk for onset.

Timing and potency of risk and subsequent onset of depression

From the developmental perspective it is critical to consider the issue of timing of risk exposure and to be able to determine the effects (potency) of risk profiles over time. From the timing perspective the potency of risk may vary. The association between increasing levels of sex hormones, tanner stage three and increased incidence of depression during this period of rapid physical change is an example of developmental timing effects on affective disorders.

Somewhat differently but equally important is determining the effects of risks over time. For example, are difficulties in childhood associated with affective disorders in adolescence. Answering questions of this nature requires longitudinal designs and is helped by repeated measurement of the candidate risk profile preferably determined prior to the study. Such cohort studies are few particularly developmentally sensitive (at any age) studies, which deliberately seek to determine the effects of risk factors through age related changes over the human lifespan. One partial example is that of Rueter and colleagues who demonstrated that among adolescents, persistent or escalating stressful events, such as disagreements with parents, indirectly increase the risk for internalizing disorder onset through their direct association with high or increasing symptom levels (Rueter *et al.*, 1999). These findings suggest that for many adolescents first episode major depression is a rather slow growing affair arising through the persisting interplay of family difficulties and rising levels of depressive symptoms over years. The study did not measure any other candidate risks either social or physiological therefore it is not easy to determine what the risk processes were that led to eventual disorder. The study is virtually unique in this age range for demonstrating quite clearly the interplay between family adversity and rising self-reported depressive symptoms and how there is not a clear direct impact of family disagreements in young teenagers, for the onset of major depression in late adolescence.

A second issue that can be addressed through longitudinal designs is that of changing effects of potency with time. What may be an important risk candidate with a large magnitude of effect at one time may be less so at another. There are no recorded invariate risk factors that continue to exert effects of the same potency for episodes of depression throughout the lifespan. Indeed there is considerable evidence that the role of environmental risks such as personally undesirable life events is markedly different for first compared with subsequent episodes of affective disorder in mid life (see Chapter 6 for further discussion of this potentially important issue regarding the relative contribution of the social environment to onset of recurrent episodes of unipolar depression).

Finally determining risk factors is only the first step in elucidating risk processes (Kraemer *et al.*, 1997). For example, if cortisol hypersecretion had true direct risk effects acting as a causal agent then lowering cortisol levels in high risk individuals might diminish the subsequent population incidence of first episode major depression in young people. Demonstrating that the risk factor can be altered and that this leads to a diminution in psychopathology would definitively demonstrate the causal nature of an antecedent risk factor, which exerted potent and toxic negative effects over a given period of time.

Risk mechanisms that result in affective symptoms and disorders

The depression theory literature, has for many years discussed the importance of exposure to adverse social experiences in the infant and pre-school years, as critical in the formation of a negative self-percept though that renders the individual more likely to depressive disorders in later life. The precise interpersonal mechanisms that may result in a child having a critical (I am not competent) and/or hostile (I am bad) view of itself are slowly beginning to emerge (see Chapter 2 for details of how parent–child relations influence the development of self-knowledge over the first decade of life). These potentially causal processes and mechanisms are best demonstrated through the use of experimental procedures ideally using subjects ascertained from population based studies of individuals at variable levels of putative risk for depression. The use of a challenge or demand paradigm allows for a putative risk circumstance to be manipulated to transiently alter the liability for the occurrence of depressive symptoms and/or personal dysfunction under controlled conditions. Interestingly this strategy has been used at most ages and stages of development to test a theory driven risk model of depressive onsets.

In children ecologically sensitive use of a competitive card game between two children has demonstrated that depressive responses to perceived personal failure during the game are likely to arise in the at risk child compared with the control companion (Murray *et al.*, 2001). In adolescents evoking dysphoric mood results in negative self-description about the self in those at high psychosocial risk for depression compared with controls (Kelvin *et al.*, 1999). In young adults and those in mid-life similar responses have been reported in numerous studies suggesting that mild dysphoric mood activates the existence of a latent negative schema of self description in at risk participants with a previous history of depression (Teasdale and Cox, 2001). A distinct neural substrate for mood-congruent processing biases in performance has recently been proposed suggesting that the medial and orbital prefrontal regions may play a key role in mediating the interaction between mood and cognition in affective disorder (Elliott et al., 2002).

These experimental strategies demonstrate the importance of mood related activation of self-devaluative cognitions in at risk subjects and those with a current and previous history of depression across the lifespan. They imply that some of the affective-cognitive mechanisms involved in the onset of first episode or recurrent unipolar depressions can be the same across the first four decades of life and demonstrate the importance of incorporating experimental approaches into risk research where there is sufficient confidence that a valid risk factor can be utilised to delineate the at risk group and a provocation is available to evoke the hypothesised response.

Whilst a powerful tool for delineate putative risk processes these complex approaches cannot address the issues of potency over time. To do so requires a combination of experimental and longitudinal approaches in a cohort of individuals repeatedly assessed with methods sensitive to their age and developmental status. For example, should at-risk five-year olds demonstrate the same characteristics during similar experimental manipulations at later stages in life this would provide considerable evidence for the origins of latent negative schemas arising in the pre-school years. Equally however a cohort design would be able to examine whether as individuals moved in and out of difficult life circumstances their response to such experimental challenges alters with more proximal adversities. If this were true then early childhood would not be the sole 'critical period' for the development of a key psychopathological process in some depressive disorders. As yet no such lifespan study involving a representative cohort has been reported.

Challenge tests have not been confined to investigations of social cognitive models of depression. The serotonin depletion hypothesis of depression has focussed on challenging this monoamine system to investigate this putative neurobiological risk for unipolar depression. The lowering of tryptophan in brain and peripheral tissues is associated with an increase in depressive symptoms, some memory changes and higher levels of aggressive behaviour (Bell et al., 2001). This occurs in the main in susceptible individuals including those with a past history of depression, a family history of depression or a positive response to antidepressants. Interestingly experimentally induced serotonergic depletion in normal individuals shifts affective memory bias towards negative affective valent verbal stimuli (Klaassen *et al.*, 2002) indicating a potential final common psychological pathway for the induction of negative symptoms of depression exemplified in statements such as I am hopeless. Whether this type of dietry depletion is more liable to exert effects in individuals psychosocially at risk over time is unclear. The role of different forms of prior psychosocial risks to the liability for a negative response to tryptophan depletion is not precisely known. Such information would considerably enhance our understanding of the sensitivity of those neurobiological systems that are candidates for mediating the effects of risk on the liability for unipolar depression. Challenge tests in which subjects have taken serotonin stimulating agents, such as 5-hydroxytryptamine or clomipramine, have also demonstrated indirect effects via measuring hormone responses in the periphery to these agents. Participants at risk for depression show blunted cortisol responses to these stimulations compared with controls although there can be marked individual variations in part related to the efficacy of the agent as well as to the nature of the risk that subjects were selected for (Park *et al.*, 1996; Birmaher *et al.*, 1997; Cowen, 1998; Kaufman *et al.*, 1998). These findings can be found across the lifespan from the first through to and including the sixth decade of life again indicating a potential mediating pathway for the effects of risk via neurobiological mechanisms. In adults there is neuroimaging evidence that changes in neural activity in distinct brain regions (ventral anterior cingulate, orbitofrontal cortex and caudate nucleus regions) mediate the clinical phenomena of depression and depression-related cognitive impairment following acute tryptophan depletion (Smith *et al.*, 1999). It is possible that these changes could be associated with the widespread distribution of serotonin neurons in brain pathways associated with the expression of affect and cognitive performance that underly the liability for unipolar depressions.

Whether these serotonin effects are related to environmental risks occurring in earlier life or arise in depressed subjects at different points in the lifespan remains to be demonstrated. Finally, genetic influences on the liability for moderating the serotonin response to adverse social circumstances may also be an important additive risk factor in the evolving of risk processes for subsequent depressions (Neumeister *et al.*, 2002).

These are selected examples of how experimental approaches can be use to test the role of neurobiological systems in affective disorders. The assumptions by many in this field is that they are testing a putative causal process (i.e. the serotonin depletion model) but the populations selected for study to date and the marked individual differences in published findings suggest that sensitivity to these neurobiological challenge procedures may be mediated by other features within the individual or arising from their adverse environment.

An integrated risk approach to understanding the nature of depressive disorders could be achieved by combining powerful experimental approaches to illuminate the complexities of risk processes within longitudinal designs using population based cohorts at different ages and stages of development. Such studies should have adequate measures of risk factors as well as clear cut assessments of the ranges of the clinical phenotype of interest.

Acknowledgements

This chapter was completed whilst the Author was in receipt of a Wellcome Trust Programme Grant and member of the MRC(UK) co-operative in Brain, Behaviour and Neuropsychiatry at the University of Cambridge.

References

American Psychiatric Association (1994). *Diagnostic and Statistical Manual For Mental and Behavioural Disorders.* American Psychiatric Association, Washington, DC.

Angold, A., Costello, E.J., Erkanl, A., *et al.* (1999). Pubertal changes in hormone levels and depression in girls. *Psychological Medicine*, **29**, 1043–1053.

Angold, A., Costello, E.J., and Erkanli, A. (1999). Comorbidity. *Journal of Child Psychology and Psychiatry*, **40**, 57–87.

Bell, C., Abrams, J., and Nutt, D. (2001). Tryptophan depletion and its implications for psychiatry. *British Journal of Psychiatry*, **178**, 399–405.

Birmaher, B., Kaufman, J., Brent, D.A., *et al.* (1997). Neuroendocrine response to 5-hydroxy-L-tryptophan in prepubertal children at high risk of major depressive disorder. *Archives of General Psychiatry*, **54**, 1113–1119.

Costello, E.J., Angold, A., and Keeler, G.P. (1999). Adolescent outcomes of childhood disorders: the consequences of severity and impairment. *Journal of the American Academy of Child and Adolescent Psychiatry*, **38**, 121–128.

Cowen, P.J. (1998). Back to the future: the neurobiology of major depression [editorial; comment]. *Psychological Medicine*, **28**, 253–255.

Elliott, R., Rubinsztein, J.S., Sahakian, B.J., *et al.* (2002). The neural basis of mood-congruent processing biases in depression. *Archives of General Psychiatry*, **59**, 597–604.

Feighner, J.P., Robins, E., Guze, S.B., *et al.* (1972). Diagnostic criteria for use in psychiatric research. *Archives of General Psychiatry*, **129**, 57–63.

Goodyer, I.M., Herbert, J., Secher, S., *et al.* (1997). Short term outcome of major depression: I. comorbidity and severity at presentation as predictors of persistent disorder. *Journal of the American Academy of Child and Adolescent Psychiatry*, **36**, 179–187.

Goodyer, I.M., Herbert, J., Tamplin, A., *et al.* (2000a). Recent life events, cortisol and DHEA in the onset of major depression amongst 'high risk' adolescents. *British Journal of Psychiatry*, 177, 499–504.

Goodyer, I.M., Herbert, J., Tamplin, A., *et al.* (2000b). First episode major depression in adolescents: affective, cognitive and endocrine characteristics of risk status and predictors of onset. *British Journal of Psychiatry*, 142–149.

Harrington, R.C., Fudge, H., Rutter, M., *et al.* (1991). Adult outcome of child and adolescent depression: II. risk for antisocial disorders. *Journal of the Amercian Academy of Child and Adolescent Psychiatry*, 30, 434–439.

Harris, T.O., Borsanyi, S., Messari, S., *et al.* (2000). Morning cortisol as a risk factor for subsequent major depressive disorder in adult women. *British Journal of Psychiatry*, 177, 505–510.

Kaufman, J., Birmaher, B., Perel, J., *et al.* (1998). Serotonergic functioning in depressed abused children: clinical and familial correlates. *Biological Psychiatry*, 44, 973–981.

Kelvin, R.G., Goodyer, I.M., Teasdale, J.D., *et al.* (1999). Latent negative self-schema and high emotionality in well adolescents at risk for psychopathology. *Journal of Child Psychology and Psychiatry*, 40, 959–968.

Kendler, K.S., Eaves, L.J., Walters, E.E., *et al.* (1996). The identification and validation of distinct depressive syndromes in a population-based sample of female twins. *Archives of General Psychiatry*, 53, 391–399.

Kendler, K.S. and Gardner, C.O., Jr. (1998). Boundaries of major depression: an evaluation of DSM-IV criteria. *American Journal of Psychiatry*, 155, 172–177.

Kendler, K.S. and Karkowski-Shuman, L. (1997). Stressful life events and genetic liability to major depression: genetic control of exposure to the environment? *Psychological Medicine*, 27, 539–547.

Kendler, K.S. and Roy, M.A. (1995). Validity of a diagnosis of lifetime major depression obtained by personal interview versus family history. *American Journal of Psychiatry*, 152, 1608–1614.

Klaassen, T., Riedel, W.J., Deutz, N.E., *et al.* (2002). Mood congruent memory bias induced by tryptophan depletion. *Psychological Medicine*, 32, 167–172.

Kolvin, I., Barret, L., Bhate, S., *et al.* (1991). The Newcastle depression project, diagnosis and classification. *British Journal of Psychiatry*, 159, 9–21.

Kovacs, M. (1997). The Emanuel Miller memorial lecture 1994. Depressive disorders in childhood: an impressionistic landscape. *Journal of Child Psychology and Psychiatry*, 38, 287–298.

Kraemer, H.C., Kazdin, A., Offord, D., *et al.* (1997). Coming to terms with the terms of Risk. *Archives of General Psychiatry*, 54, 337–343.

Lewinsohn, P. M., Clarke, G. N., Rohde, P., *et al.* (1994). Major depression in community adolescents: age at onset, episode duration, and time to recurrence. *Journal of the American Academy of Child and Adolescent Psychiatry*, 33, 809–818.

Murray, L., Woolgar, M., and Cooper, P. (2001). Cognitive vulnerability to depression in 5 year old children of depressed mothers. *Journal of Child Psychology and Psychiatry*, **42**, 891–899.

Neumeister, A., Konstantinidis, A., Stastny, J., *et al.* (2002). Association between Serotonin Transporter Gene Promoter Polymorphism (5HTTLPR) and behavioral responses to tryptophan depletion in healthy women with and without family history of depression. *Archives of General Psychiatry*, **59**, 613–620.

Park, S.B., Williamson, D.J., and Cowen, P.J. (1996). 5-HT neuroendocrine function in major depression: prolactin and cortisol responses to D-fenfluramine. *Psychological Medicine*, **26**, 1191–1196.

Pincus, H.A., Davis, W.W., and McQueen, L.E. (1999). 'Subthreshold' mental disorders. A review and synthesis of studies on minor depression and other 'brand names'. *British Journal of Psychiatry*, **174**, 288–296.

Rueter, M.A., Scaramella, L., Wallace, L.E., *et al.* (1999). First onset of depressive or anxiety disorders predicted by the longitudinal course of internalizing symptoms and parent-adolescent disagreements. *Archives of General Psychiatry*, **56**, 726–732.

Ryan, N. D., Puig-Antich, J., and Ambrosini, P. (1987). The clinical picture of major depression in childhood and adolescence. *Archives of General psychiatry*, **45**, 486–495.

Silberg, J., Pickles, A., Rutter, M., *et al.* (1999). The influence of genetic factors and life stress on depression among adolescent girls. *Archives of General Psychiatry*, **56**, 225–232.

Smith, K.A., Morris, J.S., Friston, K.J., *et al.* (1999). Brain mechanisms associated with depressive relapse and associated cognitive impairment following acute tryptophan depletion. *British Journal of Psychiatry*, **174**, 525–529.

Spitzer, T., Endicott, J., and Robins, E. (1978). Research diagnostic criteria: rational and reliability. *Archives of General Psychiatry*, **35**, 773–782.

Teasdale, J.D. and Cox, S.G. (2001). Dysphoria: self-devaluative and affective components in recovered depressed patients and never depressed controls. *Psychological Medicine*, **31**, 1311–1316.

WHO (1994). *ICD-10 Classification of Mental and Behavioural disorders.* WHO, Geneva.

Chapter 2

Intergenerational transmission of affective and cognitive processes associated with depression: infancy and the pre-school years

Lynne Murray and Peter Cooper

Introduction

This chapter focuses on the development of infants and pre-school children of women who experience depression in the postnatal months, and seeks to address a number of questions. First, we consider whether there is, in fact, evidence for adverse infant and child outcome that is associated specifically with maternal depression occurring in the postpartum period. Central to this issue is the question of the role of moderating influences; that is, whether any risks to child outcome that are associated with postnatal depression occur regardless of the context in which the maternal affective disorder occurs, or whether adverse outcomes associated with postnatal depression arise only in particular circumstances. Given the quasi-epidemiological nature of this initial question, it is important that studies from high and low risk samples are considered, with a focus on those that have employed representative community samples rather than ones that are clinic-based. Second, having addressed the question of whether postnatal depression is a risk factor for adverse child outcome, we consider what the mechanisms might be whereby such outcome associated with postpartum depression comes about. This more complex question of the processes whereby risk factors operate has, in the area of postnatal depression, been most often addressed in terms of the way in which risk might be mediated by particular patterns of parent–child relationship. Importantly, this involves consideration of the contribution of the infant, as well as the parent, to the nature of social interactions. Process questions also need to be considered at the level of what physiological effects might be involved, for example, in terms of the HPA axis, or of the development of prefrontal cortical regulation of affect and attention. Finally, we consider what implications the findings have for clinical practice.

The impact of postnatal depression— why a cause for concern?

The question whether postnatal depression may have adverse consequences for the offspring has arisen, not least, as a result of evidence from normative samples concerning the sensitivity of young infants to the quality of their interpersonal environment. In the first few months of life, the human infant is, in many ways, helpless, being neither independently mobile nor adept in manipulating his physical environment. It is, therefore, to the infant's great advantage that he establish relationships with others who will provide him with reliable and sensitive care. Experimental and observational evidence has accumulated over the past twenty-five years demonstrating the social and communicative abilities of very young infants, abilities that help the infant engage with their caretaker and secure their commitment. From birth the infant is 'experience expectant' (Greenough et al., 1987), shown in systematic preferences for human stimulation, for example, for face-like, rather than non-face-like forms (Morton and Johnson, 1991), or the human voice rather than non-human sounds, even when of the same pitch and intensity (Eisenberg, 1975). There is also evidence for expectancies for particular forms of responsiveness, so that when normal adult communication is experimentally disrupted infants only a few weeks old will avoid contact and become distressed (Tronick et al., 1978; Murray and Trevarthen, 1985). Not only does the infant show a readiness for certain forms of human contact, but there is also an impulse to form particular relationships rather than to engage indiscriminately in social interactions. This is shown in the rapid development of preferences for the sensory characteristics of those involved in the infant's care, some of which are even acquired in utero, such as that for the mother's voice and smell (Hepper, 2002). Infants also quickly pick up the interactional styles of their social partners and, in particular, their responsiveness (Meltzoff, 1990), with unresponsive partners being avoided in subsequent encounters (Bigelow and Birch, 1999). Over the early weeks and months distinctive patterns of interaction with familiar caretakers become well established, and the adult's role increasingly becomes one of supporting, or scaffolding, the infant's dealings with the wider environment. As well as promoting the infant's cognitive functioning, these parental interactions help to foster the development of infant affect and attention regulation, and establish particular patterns of parent–infant attachment.

The occurrence of depression is associated with a range of alterations in interpersonal contacts with infants, as well as with adults. In addition to facial expressions of sad, or sometimes hostile, affect, these include changes in the pitch, tempo and intonation of speech, as well as diminished eye contact and lowered responsiveness (Hinchcliffe *et al.*, 1971; Libert and Lewinsohn, 1973; Teasdale *et al.*, 1980; Bettes, 1988; Kaplan *et al.*, 2001). All of these changes occur in parameters to which the infant is sensitive in the early months. As well as the impact on expressive communication, there is also evidence that depression is associated with reduced perceptual functioning relevant to interactions with infants, such as the ability to discriminate different types of infant cry (Donovan *et al.*, 1998; Schuetze and Zeskind, 2001). The fact that the infant's primary environment in the early weeks and months is, in many cases, largely constituted by their mother, together with the early sensitivity to adult communication and the central role of social interactions in fostering infant psychological development, has added to the concern about the possible impact of postpartum depression on the child. Finally, the accumulating evidence from both animal as well as human studies of the role of the caretaking environment in the development of neuro-biological systems has provided further impetus to research in this area.

The epidemiology of postpartum depression

A number of epidemiological studies have found the prevalence of unipolar depression in the first few postpartum months to be around 10–15 per cent in the United Kingdom and United States (O'Hara, 1997), although this rate is increased in conditions of socioeconomic adversity, such as those found in the developing world (Cooper *et al.*, 1999). Although the annual prevalence of postpartum episodes does not appear to be higher than the same period prevalence in non-postpartum populations (Cooper *et al.*, 1988), there is some evidence for a stacking up of episodes in the first three months postpartum (Cooper *et al.*, 1991). Further, it seems that, for some women, childbirth is a particular risk factor. Thus, in a follow up of a UK community sample of primiparous women with postpartum depression, the pattern of risk for subsequent affective disorder differed depending on whether the postpartum disturbance was a first onset or a recurrence of depression: only those in whom the postpartum disorder was a first experience of depression were at raised risk for subsequent postpartum depression (Cooper and Murray, 1995). In terms of presentation, episodes of depression occurring in the postpartum months are indistinguishable from those occurring at other points in the life cycle; and nor is their course distinctive (Cooper *et al.*, 1988). Risk factors for postnatal depression are similar to those for depression in general, and most notably include the absence of confiding relationships, poor support from partners, and the presence of economic hardship (Cooper *et al.*, 1996).

Evidence for a specific association between postnatal depression and adverse infant and child outcome

The association between parental depression in general and adverse outcome in school-aged children is well established (see reviews by Cummings and Davies, 1994; Goodman and Gotlib, 1999; see Chapters 3 and 4, this volume). However, with regard to the effects of parental depression in the postnatal months, the evidence is far more limited. Regrettably, studies that have examined the associations between maternal depression and adverse child outcome in the pre-school years have not always analysed child functioning in relation to whether or not the child was exposed to maternal depression in the first few months. In addition, studies have not always used representative community samples, and the generalizability of their findings is therefore uncertain. Furthermore, children of mothers who experience depression in the postnatal months are at risk not only of exposure to subsequent maternal episodes of depression (Cooper and Murray, 1995), but also to a range of other adverse circumstances. These include exposure to co-morbid affective disorder and personality disorder (Radke-Yarrow and Klimes-Dougan, 1997; Carter *et al.*, 2001), marital conflict, and economic hardship (Cooper *et al.*, 1996), as well as paternal depression in the postnatal months (Deater-Deckard *et al.*, 1998). All of these factors are themselves associated with adverse infant and child outcomes. In evaluating the evidence for a specific risk of postnatal depression, therefore, it is important that account is taken of the presence of other adversity, as well as the timing of maternal depression itself. We summarize below the evidence on the cognitive and socioemotional functioning of infants and pre-school aged children of postnatally depressed mothers. We focus, in particular, on studies that have been conducted with representative community samples, and that have documented the course of maternal mood disorder throughout the child's lifetime.

Cognitive functioning

With regard to cognitive outcome, five prospective longitudinal studies of representative community samples have examined the effects of postnatal depression on preschool and school-aged children. Cogill and colleagues (1986) investigated a representative, North London, low-risk sample, and measured child IQ at age four using the McCarthy Scales. Children whose mothers had been depressed in the first postnatal year had significantly lower scores than both those of well women and those of mothers who had been depressed later on. This effect held true for both boys and girls. Further analysis of the results of this study, however, showed the adverse effects of postnatal depression to be reliable only in children whose mothers had a relatively low level of education (Hay and Kumar, 1995). A second London sample, from a more disadvantaged community, was also assessed at four years using the McCarthy Scales (Sharp et al., 1995). In this study, whilst girls were unaffected by postpartum depression, boys of women who had been depressed in the first year had significantly depressed IQ scores compared to both children who were exposed subsequently and children of well mothers. A follow-up of this cohort at 11 years (Hay et al., 2001), which looked specifically at the effects of exposure to depression in the first three months, found persistent adverse effects on the boys' general and performance IQ (using the WISC). Notably, this association between postnatal depression and boys' low IQ obtained when parental IQ and subsequent episodes of depression were taken into account. Three other studies, however, have failed to identify persistent cognitive deficits in children of mothers who were postnatally depressed. The first was conducted with a low risk, Cambridge (UK), sample. At nine and 18 months, children of postnatally depressed mothers (boys and girls) were more likely than well mothers' children to fail Object Concept tasks, and the boys of these women also had poorer scores than the other infants on a more general measure of cognitive functioning, the Mental Development Index of the Bayley Scales (Murray, 1992; Murray, Fiori-Cowley et al., 1996a). These findings are consistent with those from US clinic referred samples (Gamer et al., 1976; Lyons-Ruth et al., 1986). At five years, however, when the Cambridge cohort was assessed again using the McCarthy Scales, the earlier deficit for the boys of postnatally depressed women was no longer apparent, even among those from low SES families (Murray, Hipwell et al., 1996b). The second contrary finding comes from a large Bavarian community sample, also at low social risk. Assessments of cognitive functioning were made at 20 months (Griffiths Scales), and at four and six years (using the Columbia Mental Maturity Scales, and Kaufman Assessment Battery for Children (K-ABC), respectively) (Kurstjens and Wolke, 2001).

No adverse effects of postnatal depression per se were evident, although it was found that, for male children who were either from low SES families or who were at high neonatal risk, when postnatal episodes were followed by subsequent depression, poor Achievement Scores on the K-ABC at six years were evident. These findings are remarkably consistent with those of a recent large National (US) Maternal and Child Health survey reported by Petterson and Burke-Albers (2001). In this study, two waves of assessment were conducted. The first involved assessment of maternal depression in the year of the child's birth, and the second, at three years, involved reassessment of maternal mood and administration of the Denver Developmental Screening Test. Chronic depression (i.e. high symptom scores at both time points) was associated with substantially poorer child cognitive outcome. There was, however, also an effect, albeit a smaller one, of depression at time one only. In this study, the interaction between severity of maternal depression and family income was also an important determinant of child cognitive outcome. In cases where depression was severe, child cognitive development was negatively affected regardless of income; whereas for moderately depressed mothers only children in poor families, and particularly boys, had poor performance. Taken together, the findings yielded by these diverse samples indicate that the occurrence of depression in the postnatal period does not, in itself, pose a risk for long term poor cognitive functioning in the child. Rather, it is when other risk factors are present (e.g. low maternal education or SES, poverty, or high neonatal risk), particularly in the case of boys, that the occurrence of postnatal depression is reliably associated with adverse child outcome on measures of IQ and academic attainment.

Socioemotional and behavioural outcome

The mother–child relationship

In late infancy one of the most frequently assessed outcomes in relation to maternal depression in the postpartum months is the quality of the infant's attachment to the mother. A metaanalysis by Martins and Gaffan (2000) of seven UK and US studies that assessed children of depressed and well mothers up to age three showed a reduced likelihood of security in index children, and a corresponding raised incidence of avoidant and disorganized insecure attachments. In addition, although not measuring attachment directly, there have been findings of reduced responsiveness to maternal communication in children of postnatally depressed mothers in studies in which direct observations have been made of mother–child interactions. Thus, Stein and colleagues (1991), conducting home based observations at

19 months in the course of a longitudinal study of a representative UK sample, reported the infants of postnatally depressed women to show less shared emotion with their mothers and more anger than control group infants. While this pattern of infant behaviour was particularly evident in cases where the mother was still depressed, the effect was also present in relationships where the mother's depression had remitted, particularly where there was a high degree of marital conflict. A similar profile of less responsive engagement with the mother was found in children of postnatally depressed mothers in a follow up at five years of the low risk Cambridge sample studied by Murray and colleagues. In this case, the relationship impairments in the index group obtained even when controlling for current and chronic maternal depression, marital conflict and the quality of the mother's current behaviour towards the child. The association between postnatal depression and reduced child responsiveness was, in fact, wholly mediated by the development of insecure patterns of attachment in infancy which, in this population, were principally of the avoidant type (Murray et al., 1999). It is worth noting that these two studies' findings are remarkably similar to those reported by Cox and colleagues (1987). In this latter study, children whose mothers had experienced persistent depression up to two years postpartum but had recovered when they were followed up six months later, showed residual diminished responsiveness towards their mother, despite improvements in maternal communication.

Maternal reports

In order to assess the general behavioural and socioemotional adjustment of young children of postnatally depressed mothers, a number of studies have used maternal reports of child behavioural difficulties. Using an age-adjusted version of the Behaviour Screening Questionnaire (BSQ: Richman and Graham, 1971), an association between the occurrence of postnatal depression and behaviour problems in late infancy (18 months) was found by Murray (1992). These problems principally comprised difficulties in behavioural regulation (e.g. sleep disturbance, separation difficulties, temper tantrums). Similarly, Cicchetti and colleagues (Cicchetti et al., 1998), studying a low risk sample that included a high proportion of women who had been depressed since childbirth, found raised child behaviour problem scores at 20 months on the Child Behaviour Checklist to be associated with the occurrence of maternal depression in the child's life time, although not with current symptoms. In this sample, the relationship between maternal depression and child behaviour disturbance was mediated by general contextual risk. In relation to preschool aged children, Ghodsian Zajicek and Wolkind (1984) monitored the mental state of a London community sample of postpartum women at intervals over 42 months. Depression at four months, as well as at 14 months, was associated with maternal reports of child behaviour problems (BSQ) at 42 months, but only the effects of 14 month depression were significant when current maternal mental state was taken into account. Caplan and colleagues (1989) similarly investigated maternal reports of child behaviour at four years in a community sample of North London women followed up from pregnancy. In addition to the impact of current depression, postnatal episodes showed some link with reports of increased child disturbance, but this latter association was principally accounted for by chronic family difficulties associated with the disorder (marital conflict and paternal psychiatric history). The importance of chronic problems, including chronic depression, is similarly suggested by their association with a substantial increase in maternal reports of significant child behaviour problems at five years in the high-risk US sample of children studied by Alpern and Lyons-Ruth (1993). Nevertheless, there was some indication in this study that early maternal depression, in the absence of current symptoms, was associated with child anxiety. Further evidence for a link between postnatal episodes and poor child outcome is provided by the study of Wrate and colleagues (1985) of a Scottish community sample: postpartum depressive episodes of relatively short duration (one month) were associated with maternal reports of child behaviour problems at three years, even when controlling for current and recent depression. In this study, neither protracted postnatal episodes, nor later occurrences of depression, were associated with later child problems. The authors suggest that this somewhat counter-intuitive finding may be explained by the fact that the mothers with brief episodes were particularly anxious about their role as mother, whereas those with more chronic disorder had general preoccupations not specifically focussed on the child. Their finding is, in fact, consistent with that of a recent study of a large Australian community sample, on whom serial assessments of maternal mood were made from pregnancy to five years postpartum, when child behaviour disturbance was also assessed (Brennan et al., 2000). Where the maternal affective disturbance was of moderate severity, low maternal mood at both six months and five years was associated with elevated reports child behaviour problems. However, where this disturbance was severe, only current depressive symptoms were relevant to child outcome. Finally, in the study of Murray and colleagues, maternal reports of child behaviour problems at age five (which were strongly correlated with paternal reports) showed a significant association with postnatal depression, even when account was taken of recent and chronic episodes and the presence of marital conflict (Murray et al., 1999).

Taken together, these studies of the mother–child relationship and maternal reports of child behaviour problems at home indicate, not surprisingly, that the occurrence of chronic depressive disorder, particularly in the context of general adversity, poses the principal risk for poor child outcome. Nevertheless, there is consistent evidence, even from small studies, suggestive of behaviour difficulties in children of mothers who were depressed in the first postnatal year, but who had remitted by the time of the child assessment. The findings of reduced child responsiveness to maternal communications, despite the mother's recovery, and its possible links to earlier insecure, avoidant, attachment, further suggests that the way the mother–child relationship develops in the postpartum months is important in understanding the evolution of adverse outcomes.

Child functioning assessed independently of maternal reports: adjustment to school

The transition to school is a useful context within which to examine child functioning since it places demands on the child's personal resources, thereby elucidating any vulnerability. Since it is a normative event, it also allows comparison between children. Four studies have examined the adjustment to school of children whose mothers were depressed in the first postpartum year. Alpern and Lyons-Ruth (1993) examined by means of teacher reports the adjustment of five-year old children of low-income families. As they had found with child behaviour at home, recent and chronic maternal depression was, as expected, linked to raised rates of teacher-reported behaviour problems. Notably, however, children who had been exposed to depression by 18 months, but not those exposed at five years, were more withdrawn and anxious than children whose mothers were well. Similar findings have been reported by Essex and colleagues (Essex et al., 2001). In this prospective study of a representative, low risk Midwestern US community sample of children, teacher reports at six years showed significant effects of the timing of the child's exposure to depression. Children who had initially been exposed during their first year had high rates of comorbid internalizing and externalizing symptoms. First exposure to maternal depression beyond infancy, by contrast, only increased the risk of externalizing problems (a finding confined to girls). Notably, these associations were not altered when the chronicity of maternal depression was taken into account. Teacher reports were also examined in the study of Murray and colleagues (Sinclair and Murray, 1998). Family social class and child gender had the most pervasive effects on adjustment, with middle class children and girls being rated more favourably in terms of general school readiness and their persistence and freedom from distractibility in classroom activities. As in the studies of Alpern and Lyons-Ruth, and Essex and colleagues, recent maternal depression was related to more immature and dysregulated behaviour, but associations were also found between disruptive behaviour in boys (antisocial and hyperactive symptoms) and postnatal episodes, particularly in the context of low SES. Girls of postnatally depressed mothers, by contrast, were seen by their teachers to have low rates of behavioural disturbance. Direct observation of the children in school, however, showed both boys and girls of postnatally depressed mothers demonstrated low levels of creative play, and to be relatively unresponsive to the positive approaches of other children (Murray et al., 1999), effects that obtained when recent depression and marital conflict were taken into account. Notably, when self-cognitions were assessed in this sample in the context of mild stress (the threat of losing a competitive game with a peer), children who had been exposed to maternal depression—in most cases in the postnatal months—were more likely than non-exposed children to show evidence of depressive thinking (hopelessness, pessimism, self-denigration), even when controlling for the effects of recent and current maternal depression and the current quality of the mother's interactions with the child (Murray et al., 2001). Finally, in a small sample that included clinic referred women, Wright and colleagues (Wright et al., 2000) reported five- to eight-year old children of mothers who had experienced depression between 3 and 30 months to have more adverse outcome than children of well mothers on teacher reports of adjustment, especially on measures of aggression and poor peer relationships, even when controlling for current symptoms.

In spite of some variability in the findings, together these studies suggest that, while chronic family difficulties and current depressive symptoms in the mother are associated with raised rates of externalizing problems in children, depression in the postnatal period may be associated with an increased risk of child internalizing and anxious behaviour and the occurrence of depressive cognitions.

Mediating mechanisms

The role of maternal interactions

With regard to the central question of the way in which any adverse effects of postnatal depression on child outcome may be brought about, we turn to consider the role of early social interactions. Strikingly, the research in this area has shown that interaction patterns in the context of postnatal depression vary according to the presence or absence of additional risk factors in much the same way as does child outcome, lending support to the view that these interactions are likely to play a key role in mediating the adverse effects of the disorder. Thus, the seminal work in the 1980s by Field, Cohn and Tronick, and their colleagues (Field, 1984; Field *et al.*, 1985, 1988; Cohn *et al.*, 1986), largely conducted with populations living in conditions of high adversity, showed systematic, marked differences between groups of depressed and well women in the first six months, principally when observed during relatively brief, structured face-to-face interactions. Thus, instead of the normal pattern of responsiveness in which the parent shows contingent imitation and elaboration of infant expressions and gestures, adjusting the timing and form of response according to the infant's state of attention and affect (Brazelton *et al.*, 1974; Stern *et al.*, 1977; Trevarthen, 1979; Papousek and Papousek, 1987; Jaffe *et al.*, 2001), the depressed mothers in these samples were generally insensitive, the form of insensitivity varying from extremes of intrusive and hostile communication on the one hand, to flat, withdrawn and disengaged behaviour on the other. In turn, the infants of depressed mothers had high rates of distress and were prone to avoid contact. While subsequent research with less disadvantaged samples failed to identify these extreme deviations in the contacts between depressed mothers and their infants (e.g. Stein *et al.*, 1991; Campbell *et al.*, 1995; Murray, Fiori-Cowley *et al.*, 1996a), more subtle deficits have been found, including a reduction in depressed mothers' sensitivity to infant cues (Murray *et al.*, 1993, Murray, Fiori-Cowley *et al.*, 1996a), particularly in cases where there was also marital conflict (Stein *et al.*, 1991) and in women whose early depression persisted (Campbell *et al.*, 1995).

(a) The role of social interactions in cognitive development

There are a number of ways in which the more problematic features of depressed mothers' interactions with their infants may impair infant and child cognitive functioning (Murray *et al.*, 1993, Murray, Hipwell *et al.*, 1996b). First, the absence of contingent responsiveness is likely to be important because it reduces experiences that foster infant instrumental learning abilities (see Papousek and Papousek, 1997). Thus, micro-analytic observational studies of parent– infant interactions in normal samples have shown how parental behaviour that is sensitively responsive to, or contingent on, that of the infant in the early months is associated with the development of a generalized expectancy for predictive relations between self-generated behaviour and environmental events (Lewis and Goldberg, 1969). Indeed, when the contingent quality of adult behaviour with the infant is experimentally disrupted, the infant's subsequent performance in learning tasks is impaired (Dunham and Dunham, 1990). This kind of parental responsiveness is also likely to be important in promoting the infant's capacity for sustained attention. This is particularly evident in early interactions in the parental technique of 'theme and variation', in which adult behaviours are repeated during times of sustained mutual engagement, and changes introduced when infant attention threatens to flag (Brazelton et al., 1974; Stern et al., 1977; Papousek and Papousek, 1987; Jaffe et al., 2001). Observational studies have shown such interactions predict infant persistence in mastery motivation tasks (Yarrow et al., 1984), as well as efficient habituation (Ruddy and Bornstein, 1982). In addition, in experimental manipulations that either enhance (e.g. through encouraging parental imitation of the infant (Field, 1977)) or interfere with the contingent nature of parental engagement (e.g. by means of delayed video feedback (Murray and Trevarthen, 1985; Bigelow and Birch, 1999; Nadel et al., 1999)), infant attention is, correspondingly, either sustained, or else disrupted. The longer term importance of the infant's ability to sustain attention, and thus register and process information effectively, is reflected in the findings that attentional measures are particularly robust predictors of IQ in later childhood (Slater, 1995). In addition to their role in regulating infant attention and promoting associative learning, parental contacts that are sensitively attuned to infant cues serve the function of helping to regulate the infant's affective state (Brazelton et al., 1974; Tronick and Gianino, 1986; Tronick, 1989). This is particularly relevant to subsequent emotional and behavioural adjustment (see below), but it is also likely to be important for infant cognitive functioning. Thus, dysregulated affect is likely both to impair attention, and, as studies by Fagen and colleagues have shown, to disrupt information retrieval (Fagen et al., 1985; Singer and Fagen, 1992). Finally, a specific role of parental imitation has been proposed (Meltzoff, 1990; Murray, Hipwell et al., 1996b; Gergely, 1996) in terms of its theoretical relation to more socialcognitive capacities, including the ability to make self-other distinctions and perceive the intentional nature of others' behaviour, both of which underlie theory of mind skills.

(b) The role of early interactions in socioemotional and behavioural adjustment

There is some stability in individual differences in emotional expressiveness and reactivity from the early weeks through the first year that appears relatively independent of parenting (e.g. in terms of the amount of crying (St James-Roberts and Plewis, 1996)). However, capacities concerned with the self-regulation of behavioural and emotional states, which are key to subsequent good adjustment (Kochanska et al., 1998; Degangi et al., 2000;

Kochanska *et al.*, 2000), develop gradually (Dawson and Ashman, 2000; Posner and Rothbart, 2000), and appear more sensitive to parental intervention (Sameroff and Emde, 1989). Three ways in which parental interaction difficulties associated with depression may impede such development can be proposed. First, Field (1995) has suggested a contagion effect whereby infants show increased sad affect and distress through modelling their mothers' depressed behaviour. This suggestion is consistent with the high levels of matching of negative emotional expressions in depressed mother–infant interactions (Field *et al.*, 1990). A second possibility is that the hostile and intrusive or coercive behaviour that is particularly characteristic of depressed mothers (especially those living in conditions of marked adversity) may act directly to bring about infant distress and behavioural dysregualtion. Thus, Murray *et al.* (1996) found in a micro-analytic analysis of face-to-face interactions between depressed and well mothers and their infants that times when infant behaviour became disorganized, including distress and avoidance of contact, were systematically related to the mother's having just negated the infant's experience, usually through intrusive or hostile interventions. Support for this hypothesis derives from findings in samples of older children that the occurrence of disruptive behaviour disorders is associated with parental hostility and coercive control (Hill, 2002). Third, as the work of Tronick, and of Jaffe and Beebe, and their colleagues has shown, infants of postnatally depressed mothers may fail to gain experience of the reparation of breakdown in communication (Tronick and Gianino, 1986; Tronick, 1989; Jaffe *et al.*, 2001), as is the case for older children whose mothers are depressed (Jameson *et al.*, 1997). Thus, in normal interactions in the first few months mother and infant repeatedly shift from miscoordinated to coordinated states, the parent supporting and scaffolding the infant's immature capacities to regulate his own behaviour and affect (e.g. by reducing stimulation when the infant is over-aroused, or soothing when the infant shows distress). But if the parent is either withdrawn and disengaged, or else causes extreme distress and avoidance in the infant through aggressive interactions, opportunities for the infant to retrieve a state of equilibrium are more limited. Empirical support for the importance for later adjustment of parental strategies that promote early self-regulation has emerged both from research into the predictors of secure attachment (Isabella and Belsky, 1991; Jaffe *et al.*, 2001) and the study of the development of sleep cycles (Wolke *et al.*, 1995). It is notable that both attachment and sleep cycles are compromised in the context of postnatal depression.

In addition to the impact interaction difficulties, such as those described above, may have on observable infant behaviour, there is accumulating evidence of effects at the level of brain activity. In two series of studies, conducted by Dawson and colleagues and Field and colleagues, EEG recordings have been taken from children of postnatally depressed mothers. These have consistently shown reduced left frontal activation from the age of one to three months (Aaron-Jones *et al.*, 1997), through to six (Field *et al.*, 1995) and 15 months (Dawson *et al.*, 1997, 1999). This pattern of activation, also observed in adults experiencing depression (Schaffer *et al.*, 1983; Henrigues and Davidson, 1990), has been observed in infants of depressed mothers from both low and high risk samples. Further, it shows systematic associations with the severity of the maternal disorder, and is not accounted for by prenatal depression (Dawson *et al.*, 1997). Indeed, the authors argue that the association between reduced left frontal activation and maternal depression is mediated by the infant's experience of interaction with the mother, particularly by her non-contingent (Dawson *et al.*, 1997; Dawson, 1999) and withdrawn behaviour (Diego *et al.*, 2001). Despite this, by 13–15 months, the differences between index and control infants in frontal activity are not confined to periods when the infant is interacting with the mother, but extend to both baseline conditions and even positive interactions with an unfamiliar stranger (Dawson *et al.*, 1999).

Genetic and prenatal influences

Not only might the infant's development be influenced by the depressed mother's behaviour during social interactions, but there may also be genetic and prenatal influences on the infant associated with postnatal depression that have a bearing on poor child outcome. There is some evidence that genetic influences may be important in the occurrence of postnatal depression itself, particularly for severe, psychotic, forms (Craddock, 2000). There is also evidence consistent with the idea that genetic risk for depression in childhood may be greater in offspring of women who experience postnatal, rather then later, episodes: thus, the rate of major depression in the adolescent children of parents who themselves had early onsets of the disorder (aged under 20) is considerably greater than that in offspring of parents with later onsets (Weissman *et al.*, 1988). Caution is required when considering this line of reasoning, however, since early onset of depression in the mother is likely to be confounded with the timing of the child's exposure to the disordered environment associated with its occurrence. Indeed, in the study of Murray and colleagues in which women with a history of depression prior to childbirth, but no postnatal episodes, were compared with both well controls and postpartum depressed women and their infants, the former group, unlike the latter, did not differ from the controls either in terms of the quality of interactions in the postnatal months or in the outcome of the infants at 18 months (Murray, 1992; Murray *et al.*,

1993). These findings are consistent with those of Carter and colleagues (2001). Even if genetic mechanisms do not account directly for transmission of disorder, it is possible that they may be relevant in terms of the heritability of particular temperamental characteristics such as negative affectivity (Plomin *et al.*, 1993) or behavioural inhibition (Cherny *et al.*, 1994). However, the research on links between postnatal depression and difficult infant temperament has, in general, been neither prospective, nor had a behavioural genetic design. Thus, while it is the case that links between postnatal depression and difficult infant temperament have consistently been reported (see review by Beck, 1996), it is not clear whether such child temperament differences arise from genetic risk, or from exposure, either in pregnancy or subsequently, to adverse environmental influences. The possibility that the early parental environment may amplify any signs of difficult infant temperament is suggested by one prospective study by Hart and colleagues (Hart *et al.*, 1999). They found that the way in which infant behaviour developed over the first few weeks was predicted by initial maternal perceptions which, in the case of depressed mothers, were more negative than those of infant assessors.

With regard to other prenatal influences on the infant, maternal anxiety and stress in pregnancy, both of which are predictive of postnatal depression (Cooper *et al.*, 1996), are also associated with impaired uterine blood flow (Glover, 1997), and elevated foetal heart rate (Emory *et al.*, 1983). Similarly, the level of prenatal maternal cortisol, which is raised in the context of maternal anxiety, is predictive of that found in the foetus (Glover *et al.*, 1998). The latter finding is consistent with those of animal studies showing elevated basal levels of corticosterone in both rat (Fameli *et al.*, 1994) and non-human primate offspring (Clarke *et al.*, 1994) prenatally exposed to stress. Notably, there is evidence for continuity in patterns of heart rate and activity from foetus to neonate, and even older infants in terms of temperament (DiPietro *et al.*, 1996), blood pressure (Korner *et al.*, 1980) and stress response to inoculation at two and six months (Ramsey and Lewis, 1995). Evidence that the behaviour of infants born to antenatally depressed mothers may already be compromised at birth comes from a study in which one-day old infants of depressed women in a low socioeconomic status United States sample were found to be less responsive, and to have poorer motor tone and activity than infants of well mothers, in spite of being comparable in terms of gestational age, birthweight and perinatal variables (Abrams *et al.*, 1995).

Neonatal and infant vulnerability, whether genetic in origin, or arising from the effects of an adverse intrauterine environment associated with maternal depression, may either bear a direct relation to adverse child outcome, or it may render the infant and developing child more vulnerable to the adverse effects of poor parenting and other environmental stressors (Goodman and Gotlib, 1999; Rutter, 2000; this volume). In addition, it is important to note that difficult neonatal and infant behaviour may place the child at risk by virtue of its effects on parenting. Thus, while the studies outlined above on social interactions have focussed on the role played by parents in influencing infant emotional and cognitive processes, parent–infant relationships are bi-directional (Sameroff, 1975) and individual differences in infant behaviour may make a substantial contribution to the nature of interactions that take place. Poor infant motor control, for example, has been found to impair the infant's capacity to make eye-to-eye contact, and thus reduces opportunities for social engagement (van Wulften-Palthe and Hopkins, 1993). Furthermore, both experimentally arranged infant unresponsiveness (Murray and Trevarthen, 1986), and parental perceptions of difficult infant behaviour (Pauli-Pott *et al.*, 2000) have been found to be associated with adults becoming more hostile and less sensitive. Although, as has been noted above, such difficult neonatal behaviour may occur by virtue of risks associated with the maternal mood disorder, it can also arise quite independently of such risks. In such cases the effects on parental experience may still be substantial. Indeed, in the prospective study of Murray and colleagues, difficult behaviour (poor motor control) in neonates of mothers at both high and low risk for depression, substantially increased the risk of an onset of the maternal mood disorder within the subsequent two months (Murray, Stanley *et al.*, 1996c).

The relative contributions of infant and maternal factors to eventual child outcome

The question of how maternal behaviour and infant characteristics may combine to bring about the adverse outcomes associated with postnatal depression has received little research attention. As has been outlined above, in high risk samples, there is an increased likelihood of compromised foetal and neonatal functioning that may place the child directly at risk for poor outcome, as well as compounding further already disadvantageous patterns of parenting. However, there is evidence, even within groups of high risk infants, that adverse patterns of parenting that occur independently of infant risk mediate eventual poor child outcome; these include the links between neonatal irritability and insecure attachment (Van den Boom, 1995), low birth weight and impaired cognitive functioning (Poehlmann and Fiese, 2001), and continuity in behavioural inhibition (Kagan, 1998). In the case of low risk samples of healthy infants, the balance of influence is likely to shift further towards parental influences. Indeed, evidence from the Cambridge longitudinal low risk sample studied by Murray and colleagues showed little in the way of a direct influence of early infant characteristics on eventual child outcome. In this study, in which serial observations were made of both mother–infant interactions and infant behaviour assessed independently of the mother, it was poor early maternal responsiveness to infant cues, and a failure to engage the infant's attention in the interaction in the early postpartum months, that predicted poor cognitive functioning at 18 months; and it was these maternal factors that mediated the adverse impact of maternal depression on boys' poor performance (Murray *et al.*, 1993, Murray, Hipwell *et al.*, 1996*b*). Similarly, at five years, even though cognitive performance had generally picked up for children of postnatally depressed mothers in this sample, there was evidence of a long term effect of adverse early interactions on child outcome. Thus, children exposed to markedly unresponsive maternal behaviour in the postpartum months, who became avoidant and withdrawn in their interactions with their mother, showed poor cognitive performance at 18 months that continued to five years. Again, this impact of early interactions with the mother was not explained by independently assessed infant characteristics (Murray, Hipwell *et al.*, 1996*b*).

With regard to child behavioural and emotional functioning in this sample, similar conclusions could be drawn regarding the relatively greater importance of early maternal over infant behaviour for eventual child outcome. Somewhat different pathways from those described above relevant to poor functioning in later childhood were suggested. Again, using observations of the infant assessed independently of the mother, as well as assessments of mother–infant interactions, depressed mothers' early hostility and coercive control, which initially occurred quite independently of infant characteristics, were predictive of dysregulated attention and emotional functioning in the infant at nine months. Having once been set up, these infant difficulties were themselves associated with later disruptive behaviour symptoms, but they also placed the child at risk by eliciting further negative parenting (Morrell and Murray, 2002).

Clinical implications

The conclusion that, whatever their source, marked disturbances in the interactions between depressed mothers and their infants may set in train processes that lead to long term adverse child functioning raises important considerations concerning clinical interventions. There are consistent findings, as noted above, that depressed mothers' infants become dysregulated, withdraw from difficult interactions with their mothers, and then persist in this style of behaviour in relation both to unfamiliar non-depressed adults (Field *et al.*, 1988; Martinez *et al.*, 1996), and to their own mothers later on, despite maternal recovery from the affective disorder (Cox *et al.*, 1987; Stein *et al.*, 1991; Murray *et al.*, 1999). Moreover, the evidence from the studies conducted by Field and colleagues (1988) and Murray and colleagues (Morrell and Murray, 2002) suggests that this process of generalization to other relationships and situations is initiated within the first 6–9 months. These findings suggest, therefore, that it might be important during this period to provide the infant with consistent experience of other relationships that are free from interaction disturbance. Several lines of evidence suggest that fathers could play an important role in this regard. First, there is experimental evidence which demonstrates that infants will seek out contingently responsive partners rather than unresponsive ones when both options are available (Bigelow and Birch, 1999). Second, studies show that infants of depressed mothers respond positively during interactions with their well fathers (Hossain *et al.*, 1994). Third, it has been shown that the quality of infant attachment to the father is independent of that to the mother (Steele *et al.*, 1996). Taken together these lines of evidence suggest that fathers, if reliably available, could be important in buffering the adverse effects of maternal postnatal depression, as has been found for maternal depression occurring later on (Hops *et al.*, 1987; Conrad and Hammen, 1989). Similarly, it has been found that if the infant has become familiar with other caregivers in the early months, such as child-minders or day care nurses, generalization of the avoidance shown towards the mother is less likely to occur in interactions with these people (Pelaez-Nogueras *et al.*, 1994). While the longer term protective effects of other relationships have not been directly investigated in the context of unipolar depression, two studies have produced relevant findings. First, Cohn and colleagues (1990) note that the association between maternal depression and adverse mother–infant interactions was moderated by maternal employment, with better engagement occurring in cases where the mother was not based at home full time. Second, it is worth noting that, in the study of women admitted to hospital when experiencing bipolar postpartum episodes, infants of mothers whose caretaking was most severely affected by the disorder, and who were therefore cared for by nursing staff, showed no adverse outcome associated with the maternal episode at 12 months (Hipwell *et al.*, 2000).

There have been a number of treatment trials in the context of postnatal depression, some focussing on the mother alone, and others that encompass the mother–infant relationship. It is now well established that brief psychological treatments directed at maternal mood disorder are effective in bringing about rapid maternal remission (Holden *et al.*, 1989; Appleby *et al.*, 1997; Cooper *et al.*, 2002; O' Hara, 2000). Despite this evidence, it is unclear whether recovery from the maternal depression per se is of benefit to child developmental progress. Challenges to effecting change in the mother–infant relationship include not only the maternal difficulties, but also the fact that infants retain their memory for distinctive communication styles, and bring expectancies to interactions based on their previous experience that may make it hard to shift their negative responses to a previously insensitive mother. The treatment studies that have addressed mother–infant problems have taken a variety of forms, including focussed parenting support and interaction guidance, dynamic psychotherapy and massage therapy (Gelfand *et al.*, 1996; Field, 1997; Onozawa *et al.*, 2001; Murray *et al.*, 2002). While these programmes have sometimes been able to bring about short term improvements in mother–infant interactions (Field, 1997; Onozawa *et al.*, 2001), this has not always been the case, particularly in low risk samples (Gelfand *et al.*, 1996; Murray *et al.*, 2002); and while maternal reports of difficulties, including those concerning child behaviour, have shown medium term benefits, infant attachment and cognitive outcomes have not been improved (Gelfand *et al.*, 1996; Murray *et al.*, 2002).

An attractive prospect would be to prevent the occurrence of postpartum depression and thereby prevent the disturbed mother–infant interactions and the associated adverse infant outcome. This possibility has yet to be tested empirically. A major obstacle to advancing along these lines is that it depends on being able to identify women at antenatal risk for the development of postpartum mood disorder and being able to intervene successfully. Although some progress has been made in the development of methods for antenatal identification of antenatal vulnerability (Cooper *et al.*, 1996), prediction is, at best, only modestly successful. A more significant impediment is the fact that, despite several controlled trials of preventive interventions, there is, to date, no convincing evidence that these have an impact on the rate of postpartum depressive disorder (Stamp *et al.*, 1995; Buist *et al.*, 1999; Brugha *et al.*, 2000; Elliott *et al.*, 2000). Until such evidence is produced, there are no grounds for concentrating therapeutic efforts on prevention, and it is far more appropriate to focus on treatment of the maternal disorder and support for other carers.

Conclusions

There is evidence from epidemiological studies that postnatal depression is associated with risks to child outcome. The risk for poor cognitive functioning associated with postnatal depression occurs principally when other risk factors are present (e.g. high levels of socioeconomic adversity, low birth weight, and subsequent maternal episodes), as does that for externalizing behaviour problems. However, the increased likelihood of insecure child attachment, and the occurrence of internalizing symptoms in the children of postnatally depressed mothers, appear to occur independently of the impact of other adversity. More limited evidence is available concerning the processes leading to poor child outcome. A combination of genetic risk and adverse intrauterine influences may increase infant vulnerability, both directly, and via the impact of difficult infant behaviour on parents. However, adverse patterns of parenting, whether elicited by neonatal and infant behaviours, or occurring independently, are likely to play a major role in bringing about poor child outcome. Attempts to change parental interactions and improve the outcome for children of postnatally depressed mothers have met with limited success, and an important therapeutic strategy may well be to enhance the role of other caregivers.

References

Aaron Jones, N., Field, T., Fox, N.A., Lundy, B., and Davalos, M. (1997). EEG activation in 1-month-old infants of depressed mothers. *Development and Psychopathology*, 9, 491–505.

Abrams, S.M., Field, T., Scafidi, F., and Prodromidis, M. (1995). Newborns of depressed mothers. *Infant Mental Health Journal*, 16(3), 233–239.

Alpern, L. and Lyons-Ruth, K. (1993). Preschool children at social risk: chronicity and timing of maternal depressive symptoms and child behavior problems at school and at home. *Development and Psychopathology*, 5, 371–387.

Appleby, L., Warner, R., Whitton, A., and Garagher, B. (1997). A controlled study of fluoxetine and cognitive-behavioural counselling in the treatment of postnatal depression. *British Medical Journal*, 314, 932–936.

Beck, C.T. (1996). A meta-analysis of the relationship between postpartum depression and infant temperament. *Nursing Research*, 45(4), 22230.

Bettes, B.A. (1988). Maternal depression and motherese: temporal and intonatinal features. *Child Development*, 59, 1089–1096.

Bigelow, A.E. and Birch, S.A.J. (1999). The effects of contingency in previous interactions on infants' preference for social partners. *Infant Behavior and Development*, 22(2), 257–262.

Brazelton, T.B., Koslowski, B., and Main, M. (1974). The origins of reciprocity: the early mother-infant interaction. In M. Lewis and L.A. Rosenblum (Eds.), *The Effects of the Infant on its Caregiver*. Wiley, New York.

Brennan, P.A., Hammen, C., Andersen, M.J., Bor, W., Najman, J.M., and Williams, G.M. (2000). Chronicity, severity, and timing of maternal depressive symptoms: relationships with child outcomes at age 5. *Developmental Psychology*, **36**(6), 759–766.

Brugha, T., Wheatley, S., Taub, N.A., Culverwell, A., Friedman, T., Kirwan, P., Jones, D.R., and Shapiro, D.A. (2000). Pragmatic randomized trial of antenatal intervention to prevent post-natal depression by reducing psychosocial risk factors. *Psychological Medicine*, **30**, 1273–1281.

Buist, A., Westley, D., and Hill, C. (1999). Antenatal prevention of postnatal depression. *Archives of Women's Mental Health*, **1**, 167–173.

Campbell, S.B., Cohn, J.F., and Meyers, T. (1995). Depression in first-time mothers: mother-infant interaction and depression chronicity. *Developmental Psychology*, **31**(3), 349–357.

Caplan, H., Cogill, S., Alexandra, H., Robson, K., Katz, R., and Kumar, R. (1989). Maternal depression and the emotional development of the child. *British Journal of Psychiatry*, **154**, 818–823.

Carter, A.S., Garrity-Rokous, F.E., Chazan-Cohen, R.C.L., and Briggs-Gowan, M.J. (2001). Maternal depression and comorbidity: predicting early parenting, attachment security, and toddler social-emotional problems and competencies. *American Academy of Child and Adolescent Psychiatry*, **40**(1), 18–26.

Cherny, S.S., Fulker, D.W., Corley, R.P., Plomin, R., and DeFries, J.C. (1994). Continuity and change in infant shyness from 14 to 20 months. *Behavior Genetics*, **24**, 365–379.

Cicchetti, D., Rogosch, F.A., and Toth, S.L. (1998). Maternal depressive disorder and contextual risk: contributions to the development of attachment insecurity and behavior problems in toddlerhood. *Development and Psychopathology*, **10**, 283–300.

Clarke, A.S., Wittwer, D.J., Abbott, D.H., and Schneider, M.L. (1994). Long-term effects of prenatal stress on HPA axis activity in juvenile rhesus monkeys. **27**, 256–269.

Cogill, S.R., Caplan, H.L., Alexandra, H., Robson, K.M., and Kumar, R. (1986). Impact of maternal postnatal depression on cognitive development of young children. *British Medical Journal*, **292**(6529), 1165–1167.

Cohn, J.F., Campbell, S.B., Matias, R., and Hopkins, J. (1990). Face-to-face interactions of postpartum depressed and nondepressed mother-infant pairs at 2 months. *Developmental Psychology*, **26**(1), 15–23.

Cohn, J.F., Matias, R., Tronick, E.Z., Connell, D., and Lyons-Ruth, K. (1986). Face-to-face interactions of depressed mothers and their infants. In Z. Tribucjm E and T. Field (Eds.), *Maternal Depression and Infant Disturbance*. Jossey-Bass, Francisco, pp. 31–46.

Conrad, M. and Hammen, C. (1989). Role of maternal depression in perceptions of child maladjustment. *Journal of Consulting and Clinical Psychology*, **57**, 663–667.

Cooper, P.J., Campbell, E.A., Day, A., Kennerly, H., and Bond, A. (1988). Non-psychotic psychiatric disorder after childbirth: a prospective study of prevalence, incidence, course and nature. *British Journal of Psychiatry*, **152**, 799–806.

Cooper, P.J. and Murray, L. (1995). The course and recurrence of postnatal depression: evidence for the specificity of the diagnostic concept. *British Journal of Psychiatry*, **166**, 191–195.

Cooper, P.J. and Murray, L. (1997). The impact of psychological treatments of postpartum depression on maternal mood and infant development. In L. Murray and P.J. Cooper (Eds.), *Postpartum Depression and Child Development*. Guilford, New York, pp. 201–220.

Cooper, P.J., Murray, L., Hooper, R., and West, A. (1996). The development and validation of a predictive index for postnatal depression. *Psychological Medicine*, **26**, 627–634.

Cooper, P.J., Murray, L., and Stein, A. (1991). Postnatal depression. In J. Seva (Ed.), *The European Handbook of Psychiatry and Mental Health*. Anthropos, Zaragos.

Cooper, P.J., Murray, L., Wilson, A., and Romaniuk, H. (2002). A controlled trial of the short and long term effect of psychological treatment of postpartum depression: I impact on maternal mood. *British Journal of Psychiatry*, (*under review*).

Cooper, P.J., Tomlinson, M., Swartz, L., Woolgar, M., Murray, L., and Molteno, C. (1999). Post-partum depression and the mother-infant relationship in a South African peri-urban settlement. *British Journal of Psychiatry*, **175**, 554–558.

Cox, A.D., Puckering, C., Pound, A., and Mills, M. (1987). The impact of maternal depression in young children. *Journal of Child Psychology and Psychiatry*, **28**(6), 917–928.

Craddock, N. (2000, September 2000). *Genetic Investigations of Puerperal Psychosis*. Paper presented at the Marce Conference, Manchester.

Cummings, E.M. and Davies, P.T. (1994). Maternal depression and child development. *Journal of Child Psychology and Psychiatry*, **35**(1), 73–112.

Dawson, G. (1999). *The Effects of Maternal Depression on Children's Emotional and Psychobiological Development*. Paper presented at the National Institutes of Health Conference on Parenting, Bethesda, MD.

Dawson, G. and Ashman, S.B. (2000). On the origins of a vulnerability to depression: the influence of the early social environment on the development of psychobiological systems related to risk for affective disorder. In C. Nelson (Ed.), *The Minnesota symposium on child psychology* (Vol. **31**,). Mahwah, New Jersey.

Dawson, G., Frey, K., Panagiotides, H., Osterling, J., and Hessl, D. (1997*a*). Infants of depressed mothers exhibit atypical frontal brain activity: a replication and extension of previous findings. *Journal of Child Psychology and Psychiatry*, **38**(2), 179–186.

Dawson, G., Frey, K., Panagiotides, H., Self, J., Hessl, D., and Yamada, E. (1997*b*). *Atypical Frontial Brain Activity in Infants of Depressed Mothers: The Role of Maternal Behavior*. Paper presented at the Poster presented at the 1997 Meeting of the Society for Research in Child Development, Washington, DC.

Dawson, G., Frey, K., Panagiotides, H., Yamada, E., Hessl, D., and Osterling, J. (1999*a*). Infants of depressed mothers exhibit atypical frontal electrical brain activity during interactions with mother and with a familiar, nondepressed adult. *Child Development*, **70**(5), 1058–1066.

Dawson, G., Frey, K., Panagiotides, H., Yamada, E., Hessl, D., and Osterling, J. (1999*b*). Infants of depressed mothers exhibit atypical frontal electrical brain activity during interactions with mother and with a familiar, nondepressed adult. *Child Development*, **70**(5), 1058–1066.

Deater-Deckard, K., Pickering, K., Dunn, J.F., Golding, J., and Team, A.L.S.O.P.A.C.S. (1998). Family structure and depressive symptoms in men preceding and following the birth of a child. *American Journal of Psychiatry*, **155**(6), 818–823.

Degangi, G.A., Breinbauer, C., Doussard Roosevelt, J., Proges, S., and Greenspan, S. (2000). Prediction of childhood problems at three years in children experiencing disorders of regulation during infancy. *Infant Mental Health Journal*, **21**(3), 156–175.

Diego, M.A., Field, T., and Hernandez-Reif, M. (2001). BIS/BAS scores are correlated with frontal EEG asymmetry in intrusive and withdrawn depressed mothers. *Infant Mental Health Journal*, **22**(6), 665–675.

DiPietro, J.A., Hodgson, D.M., and Costigan, K.A. (1996). Fetal antecedents of infant temperament. *Child Development*, **67**, 2568–2583.

Donovan, W.L., Leavitt, L.A., and Walsh, R.O. (1998). Conflict and depression predict maternal sensitivity to infant cries. *Infant Behavior and Development*, **21**(3), 505–517.

Dunham, P.J. and Dunham, F. (1990). Effects of mother-infant social interactions on infants' subsequent contingency task performance. *Child Development*, **61**, 785–793.

Eisenberg, R.B. (1975). *Auditory Competence in Early Life. The Roots of Communicative Behaviour.* University Park Press, Baltimore.

Elliott, S.A., Leverton, T.J., Sanjack, M., *et al.* (2000). Promoting mental health after childbirth: a controlled trial of primary prevention of postnatal depression. *British Journal of Clinical Psychology*, **39**, 223–241.

Emory, E., Walker, E., and Cruz, A. (1983). Fetal heart rate: II behavioral correlates. *Psychophysiology*, **19**, 680–686.

Essex, M.J., Klein, M.H., Miech, R., and Smider, N.A. (2001). Timing of initial exposure to maternal major depression and children's mental health symptoms in kindergarten. *British Journal of Psychiatry*, **179**, 151–154.

Fagen, J.W., Ohr, P.S., Fleckenstein, L.K., and Ribner, D.R. (1985). The effect of crying on long-term memory in infancy. *Child Development*, **56**, 1584–1592.

Fameli, M., Kitraki, E., and Stylianopoulou, F. (1994). Effects of hyperactivity of the maternal hypothalamic-pituitary-adrenal (HPA) axis during pregnancy on the development of the HPA axis and brain monoamines of the offspring. *International Journal of Developmental Neuroscience*, **12**, 651–659.

Field, T. (1977). Effects of early separation, interactive deficits, and experimental manipulations on infant-mother face-to-face interaction. *Child Development,* **48,** 75–771.

Field, T. (1995). Infants of depressed mothers. *Infant Behavior and Development,* **18,** 1–13.

Field, T. (1997). The treatment of depressed mothers and their infants. In L. Murray and P.J. Cooper (Eds.), *Postpartum Depression and Child Development.* Guilford, New York, pp. 221–236.

Field, T., Fox, N., Pickens, J., Nawrocki, T., and Soutullo, D. (1995). Right front EEG activation in 3- to 6 month-old infants of "depressed" mothers. *Developmental Psychology,* **31,** 358–363.

Field, T., Healy, B., Goldstein, S., and Gurthertz, M. (1990). Behavior-state matching and synchrony in mother-infant interactions of nondepressed versus depressed dyads. *Developmental Psychology,* **26**(1), 7–14.

Field, T., Healy, B., Goldstein, S., Perry, S., Bendell, D., Schanberg, S., Ximmerman, E.A., and Kuhn, C. (1988). Infants of depressed mothers show "depressed" behavior even with nondepressed adults. *Child Development,* **59,** 1569–1579.

Field, T., Sandberg, D., Garcia, R., Vega-Lahr, N., Goldstein, S., and Guy, L. (1985). Pregnancy problems, postpartum depression, and early mother-infant interactions. *Developmental Psychology,* **21**(6), 1152–1156.

Field, T.M. (1984). Early interactions between infants and their postpartum depressed mothers. *Infant Behavior and Development,* **7,** 517–522.

Gamer, E., Gallant, D., and Grunebaum, H. (1976). Children of psychotic mothers. An evaluation of 1-year-olds on a test of object permanence. *Archive of General Psychiatry,* **33,** 311–317.

Gelfand, D.M., Teti, D.M., Seiner, S.A., and Jameson, P.B. (1996). Helping mothers fight depression: evaluation of a home-based intervention program for depressed mothers and their infants. *Clinical Child Psychology,* **25**(4), 406–422.

Gergely, G. (1996). The social biofeedback theory of parental affect-mirroring. *Internal Journal of Psycho-Anal.,* **77,** 1181–1211.

Ghodsian, M., Zajicek, E., and Wolkind, S. (1984). A longitudinal study of maternal depression and child behaviour problems. *Journal of Child Psychology and Psychiatry,* **25**(1), 91–109.

Glover, V. (1997). Maternal stress or anxiety in pregnancy and emotional development of the child. *British Journal of Psychiatry,* **171,** 105–106.

Glover, V., Teixeira, J., Gitau, R., and Frisk, N. (1998). *Links Between Antenatal Maternal Anxiety and the Fetos.* Paper presented at the 11th Biennial Conference on Infant Studies, Atlanta, GA.

Goodman, S.H. and Gotlib, I.H. (1999). Risk for psychopathology in the children of depressed mothers: a developmental model for understanding mechanisms of transmission. *Psychological Review,* **106**(3), 458–490.

Greenough, W.T., Black, J.E., and Wallace, C.S. (1987). Experience and brain development. *Child Development*, **58**, 539–559.

Hart, S., Field, T., and Roitfarb, M. (1999). Depressed mothers' assessments of their neonates' behaviors. *Infant Mental Health Journal*, **20**(2), 200–210.

Hay, D.F. and Kumar, R. (1995). Interpreting the effects of mothers' postnatal depression on children's intelligence: a critique and re-analysis. *Child Psychiatry and Human Development*, **253**, 165–181.

Hay, D.F., Pawlby, S., Sharp, D., Asten, P., Mills, A., and Kumar, R.K. (2001). Intellectual problems shown by 11-year-old children whose mothers had postnatal depression. *Journal of Child Psychology and Psychiatry*, **42**(7), 871–889.

Henriques, J.B. and Davidson, R.J. (1990). Regional brain electrical asymmetrics discriminate between previously depressed and healthy control subjects. *Journal of Abnormal Psychology*, **99**, 22–31.

Hepper, P.G. (2002). Prenatal development. In A. Slater and M. Lewis (Eds.), *Introduction to Infant Development*. Oxford University Press, Oxford, pp. 39–60.

Hill, J. (2002). Biological, psychological and social processes in the conduct disorders. *Child Psychology and Psychiatry*, **43**(1), 133–164.

Hinchcliffe, M.K., Lancashire, M., and Roberts, F.J. (1971). A study of eye-contact changes in depressed and recovered psychiatric patients. *British Journal of Psychiatry*, **119**, 213–215.

Hipwell, A., Goossens, F., Melhuish, E., and Kumar, R. (2000). Severe maternal psychopathology and infant-mother attachment. *Development and Psychopathology*, **12**, 157–175.

Holden, J., Sagavsky, R., and Cox, J.L. (1989). Counselling in a general practice setting: a controlled study of health visitor intervention in the treatment of postnatal depression. *British Medical Journal*, **298**, 223–226.

Hops, H., Biglan, A., Sherman, L., Arthur, J., Friedman, L., and Osteen, V. (1987). Home observations of family interactions of depressed women. *Journal of Consulting and Clinical Psychology*, **53**, 341–346.

Hossain, Z., Field, T., Gonzalez, J., Malphurs, J., and Del Valle, C. (1994). Infants of "depressed" mothers interact better with their nondepressed fathers. *Infant Mental Health*, **15**(4), 348–357.

Isabella, R. and Belsky, J. (1991). Interactional synchrony and the origins of mother-infant attachment: a replication study. *Child Development*, **62**, 373–384.

Jaffe, J., Beebe, B., Feldstein, S., Crown, C., and Jasnow, M.D. (2001). *Rhythms of Dialogue in Infancy: Coordinated Timing in Development*. (Vol. 2). Blackwell, Massachusetts.

Jameson, P.B., Gelfand, D.M., Kulcsar, E., and Teti, D.M. (1997). Mother-toddler interaction patterns associated with maternal depression. *Development and Psychopathology*, **9**, 537–550.

Kagan, J. (1998). *Galen's Prophecy*. Westview Press, Colorado.

Kaplan, P.S., Bachorowski, J., Smoski, M.J., and Zinser, M. (2001). Role of clinical diagnosis and medication use in effects of maternal depression on infant-directed speech. *Infancy*, **2**(4), 537–548.

Kochanska, G., Murray, K.T., and Harlan, E.T. (2000). Effortful control in early childhood: continuity and change, antecedents, and implications for social development. *Developmental Psychology*, **36**(2), 220–232.

Kochanska, G., Tjebkes, T.L., and Forman, D.R. (1998). Children's emerging regulation of conduct: restraint, compliance, and internalization from infancy to the second year. *Child Development*, **69**(5), 1378–1389.

Korner, A.F., Gabby, T., and Kraemer, H.C. (1980). Relation between prenatal blood pressure and infant irritability. *Early Human Development*, **4**(1), 35–39.

Kurstjens, S. and Wolke, D. (2001). Effects of maternal depression on cognitive development of children over the first 7 years of life. *Journal of Child Psychology and Psychiatry*, **42**(5), 623–636.

Lewis, M. and Goldberg, S. (1969). Perceptual-cognitive development in infancy: a generalised expectancy model as a function of the mother-infant interaction. *Merrill-Palmer Quarterly*, **3**, 307–316.

Libert, J. and Lewinsohn, P.M. (1973). The concept of social skill with special reference to the behavior of depressed persons. *Journal of Consulting and Clinical Psychology*, **40**, 304–312.

Lyons-Ruth, K., Zoll, D., Connell, D., and Grunebaum, H.V. (1986). The depressed mother and her one year old infant. In T. Field and E. Tronick (Eds.), *Maternal Depression and Child Disturbance* Vol. **34**, Jossey-Bass, San Francisco, pp. 31–46.

Martinez, A., Malphurs, J., Field, T., Pickens, J., Uando, R., Bendell, D., Valle, C., and Messinger, D. (1996). Depressed mothers' and their infants' interactions with nondepressed partners. *Infant Mental Health Journal*, **17**(1), 74–80.

Martins, C. and Gaffan, E.A. (2000). Effects of early maternal depression on patterns of infant-mother attachment: a meta-analytic investigation. *Journal of Child Psychology and Psychiatry*, **41**(6), 737–746.

Meltzoff, A.N. (1990). Foundations for developing a concept of self: the role of imitation in relating self to other and the value of social mirroring, social modeling, and self practice in infancy. In D. Cicchetti and M. Beeghly (Eds.), *The Self in Transition: Infancy to Childhood*. University of Chicago Press, Chicago, Ill, pp. 139–164.

Morrell, J. and Murray, L. Postnatal depression and the development of conduct disorder and hyperactive symptoms in childhood: a prospective longitudinal study from 2 months to 8 years. *Journal of Child Psychology and Psychiatry*, *(under review)*.

Morton, J. and Johnson, M.H. (1991). CONSPEC and CONLERN: a two-process theory of infant face recognition. *Psychological Review*, **98**, 164–181.

Murray, L. (1992). The impact of postnatal depression on infant development. *Journal of Child Psychology and Psychiatry*, **33**, 543–561.

Murray, L., Cooper, P.J., Wilson, A., and Romaniuk, H. (2002). A controlled trial of the long term effect of psychological teatment of postpartum depression: II impact on the mother child relationship and child outcome. *British Journal of Psychiatry, (under review)*.

Murray, L., Fiori-Cowley, A., Hooper, R., and Cooper, P.J. (1996*a*). The impact of postnatal depression and associated adversity on early mother-infant interactions and later infant outcome. *Child Development*, **67**, 2512–2526.

Murray, L., Hipwell, A., Hooper, R., Stein, A., and Cooper, P.J. (1996*b*). The cognitive development of five year old children of postnatally depressed mothers. *Journal of Child Psychology and Psychiatry*, **37**, 927–935.

Murray, L., Kempton, C., Woolgar, M., and Hooper, R. (1993). Depressed mothers' speech to their infants and its relation to infant gender and cognitive development. *Journal of Child Psychology and Psychiatry*, **34**, 1083–1101.

Murray, L., Sinclair, D., Cooper, P.J., Ducournau, P., Turner, P., and Stein, A. (1999*a*). The socio-emotional development of five year old children of postnatally depressed mothers. *Journal of Child Psychology and Psychiatry*, **40**(8), 1259–1272.

Murray, L., Stanley, C., Hooper, R., King, F., and Fiori-Cowley, A. (1996*c*). The role of infant factors in postnatal depression and the mother-infant interactions. *Developmental Medicine and Child Neurology*, **38**, 109–119.

Murray, L. and Trevarthen, C. (1985). Emotional regulation of interactions between two months olds and their mother. In T.M. Field and N. Fox (Eds.), *Social Perception in Infants*. Ablex, New Jersey.

Murray, L. and Trevarthen, C. (1986). The infant's role in mother-infant communication. *Journal of Child Language*, **13**, 15–29.

Murray, L., Woolgar, M., Briers, S., and Hipwell, A. (1999*b*). The representation of family life of children of depressed and well mothers. *Social Development*, **8**(2), 179–200.

Murray, L., Woolgar, M., Cooper, P.J., and Hipwell, A. (2001). Cognitive vulnerability in five year old children of depressed mothers. *Journal of Child Psychology and Psychiatry*, **42**(7), 891–899.

Nadel, J., Carchon, I., Kervella, C., Marcelli, D., and Reserbat-Plantey, D. (1999). Expectancies for social contingency in 2-month-olds. *Developmental Science*, **2**(2), 164–173.

O'Hara, M. (1997). Introduction to postpartum depressive disorders. In L. Murray and P.J. Cooper (Eds.), *Postpartum Depression and Child Development*. Guilford, New York, pp. 3–31.

O' Hara, M., Stuart, S., Gorman, L., and Wenzel, A. (2000). Efficacy of interpersonal psychotherapy for postpartum depression. *Archives of General Psychiatry*, **57**, 1039–1045.

Onozawa, K., Glover, V., Adams, D., Modi, N., and Kumar, R.C. (2001). Infant massage improves mother-infant interaction for mothers with postnatal depression. *Journal of Affective Disorders*, **63**, 201–207.

Palaez-Nogueras, M., Field, T., Cigales, M., Gonzalez, A., and Clasky, S. (1994). Infants of depressed mothers show less "depressed" behavior with their nursery teachers. *Infant Mental Health*, 15, 358–367.

Papousek, H. and Papousek, M. (1987). Intuitive parenting: a dialectic counterpart to the infant's integrative competence. In J.D. Osofsky (Ed.), *Handbook of Infant Development* (2nd edition), Wiley, New York, pp. 669–720.

Papousek, H. and Papousek, M. (1997). Fragile aspects of early social integration. In L. Murray and P.J. Cooper (Eds.), *Postpartum Depression and Child Development*. The Guilford Press, New York, pp. 35–53.

Pauli-Pott, U., Mertesacker, B., Bade, U., Bauer, C., and Beckmann, D. (2000). Contexts of relations of infant negative emotionality to caregiver's reactivity/sensitivity. *Infant Behavior and Development*, 23, 23–39.

Petterson, S.M. and Burke-Albers, A. (2001). Effects of poverty and maternal depression on early child development. *Child Development*, 72(6), 1794–1813.

Plomin, R., Emde, R.N., Braungart, J.M., Campos, J., Corley, R., Fulker, D.W., Kagan, J., Reznick, J.S., Robinson, J., Zahn-Waxler, C., and Defries, J.C. (1993). Genetic change and continuity from fourteen to twenty months: the MacArthur longitudinal twin study. *Child Development*, 64, 1354–1376.

Poehlmann, J. and Fiese, B.H. (2001). Parent-infant interaction as a mediator of the relation between neonatal risk status and 12-month cognitive development. *Infant Behavior and Development*, 24, 171–188.

Posner, M.I. and Rothbart, M.K. (2000). Developing mechanisms of self-regulation. *Development and Psychopathology*, 12, 427–441.

Radke-Yarrow, M. and Klimes-Dougan, B. (1997). Children of depressed mothers: a developmental and interactional perspective. In S.S. Luthar and J.A. Burack (Eds.), *Developmental Psychopathology: Perspectives on Adjustment, Risk and Disorder*. Cambridge University Press, New York, pp. 374–389.

Ramsay, D.S. and Lewis, M. (1995). The effects of birth condition on infants' cortisol response to stress. *Pediatrics*, 95, 546–549.

Richman, N. and Graham, P. (1971). A behavioural screening questionnaire for use with three-year old children: preliminary findings. *Journal of Child Psychology and Psychiatry*, 12, 5–33.

Ruddy, M.G. and Bornstein, M.H. (1982). Cognitive correlates of infant attention and maternal stimulation over the 1st year of life. *Child Development*, 53(1), 183–188.

Rutter, M. (2000). Psychosocial influences: critiques, findings, and research needs. *Development and Psychopathology*, 12, 375–405.

Sameroff, A.J. (1975). Transactional models in early social relations. *Human Development*, 18(65).

Sameroff, A.J. and Emde, R.N. (1989). *Relationship Disturbances in Early Childhood: A Developmental Approach*. Basic books, New York.

Schaffer, C.E., Davidson, R.J., and Saron, C. (1983). Frontal and parietal electroencephalogram activation in depressed and nondepresed subjects. *Biological Psychiatry*, 18, 753–762.

Schuetze, P. and Zeskind, P.S. (2001). Relations between women's depressive symptoms and perceptions of infant distress signals varying in pitch, *Influence of depression on ratings of infant cries* (pp. 484–499): Lawrence Enbaum Associates.

Sharp, D., Hay, D., Pawlby, S., Schmucher, G., Allen, H., and Kumar, R. (1995). The impact of postnatal depression on boys intellectual development. *Journal of Child Psychology and Psychiatry*, **36**, 1315–1337.

Sinclair, D. and Murray, L. (1998). The effects of postnatal depression on children's adjustment to school: teacher reports. *British Journal of Psychiatry*, **172**, 58–63.

Singer, J.M. and Fagen, J.W. (1992). Negative affect, emotional expression, and forgetting in young infants. *Developmental Psychology*, **28**(1), 48–57.

Slater, A. (1995). Individual differences in infancy and later IQ. *Journal of Child Psychology and Psychiatry*, **36**, 69–112.

St James-Roberts, I. and Plewis, I. (1996). Individual differences, daily fluctuations, and developmental changes in amounts of infant waking, fussing, crying, feeding, and sleeping. *Child Development*, **67**, 2527–2540.

Stamp, G.E., Williams, A.S., and Crowther, C.A. (1995). Evaluation of antenatal and postnatal support to overcome postnatal depression: a randomized control trial. *Birth*, **22**, 138–143.

Steele, H., Steele, M., and Fonagy, P. (1996). Associations among attachment classifications of mothers, fathers, and their infants: evidence for a relationship-specific perspective. *Child Development*, **67**, 541–555.

Stein, A., Gath, D.H., Bucher, J., Bond, A., Day, A., and Cooper, P.J. (1991). The relationship between post-natal depression and mother-child interaction. *British Journal of Psychiatry*, **158**, 46–52.

Stern, D.N., Beebe, B., Jaffe, J., and Bennett, S.L. (1977). The infant's stimulus world during social interaction: a study of caregiver behaviours with particular reference to repetition and timing. In H.R. Schaffer (Ed.), *Studies in Mother-Infant Interaction*. Academic Press, London, pp. 177–202.

Teasdale, J.D., Fogarty, S.J., and Williams, J.M.G. (1980). Speech rate as a measure of short-term variation in depression. *British Journal of Social and Clinical Psychology*, **19**, 271–278.

Trevarthen, C. (1979). Communication and cooperation in early infancy: a description of primary intersubjectivity. In M.M. Bullowa (Ed.), *Before speech: The Beginning of Interpersonal Communication*. Cambridge University Press, New York, pp. 321–349.

Tronick, E., Als, H., Adamson, L., Wise, S., and Brazelton, T.B. (1978). The infant's response to entrapment between contradictory messages in face-to-face interaction. *American Academy of Child Psychiatry*, 1–13.

Tronick, E.Z. (1989). Emotions and emotional communication in infants. *American Psychologist*, **44**(2), 112–119.

Tronick, E.Z. and Gianino, A. (1986). Interactive mismatch and repair: challenges to the coping infant. *Zero to Three. National Center for Clinical Infant Programs*, **6**(3), 1–6.

van den Boom, D.C. (1995). Do first-year intervention effects endure? Follow-up during toddlerhood of a sample Dutch irritable infants. *Child Development*, **66**, 1798–1816.

van Wulfften Palthe, T. and Hopkins, B. (1993). A longitudinal study of neural maturation and early mother-infant interaction: a research note. *Journal of Child Psychology and Psychiatry*, **34**, 1031–1041.

Weissman, M.M., Wickramaratne, P., and Prusoff, B.A. (1988). Early-onset major depression in parents and their children. *Journal of Affective Disorders*, **15**, 269–277.

Wolke, D., Renate, M., Ohrt, B., and Riegel, K. (1995). The incidence of sleeping problems in preterm and fullterm infants discharged from neonatal special care units: an epidemiological longitudinal study. *Child Psychology and Psychiatry*, **36**(2), 203–223.

Wrate, R.M., Rooney, A.C., Thomas, P.F., and Cox, J.L. (1985). Postnatal depression and child development. A three-year follow-up study. *British Journal of Psychiatry*, **146**, 622–627.

Wright, C.A., George, T.P., Burke, R., Gelfand, D.M., and Teti, D.M. (2000). Early maternal depression and children's adjustment to school. *Child Study Journal*, **30**(3), 153–168.

Yarrow, L.J., MacTurk, R.H., Vietze, P.M., McCarthy, M.E., Klein, R.P., and McQuiston, S. (1984). Developmental course of parental stimulation and its relationship to mastery motivation during infancy. *Developmental Psychology*, **20**, 492–505.

Chapter 3

Unipolar depression—a lifespan perspective: 'The School Age Child'

Boris Birmaher and John Samuel Rozel

This chapter reviews the literature on the epidemiology, etiology, clinical characteristics, natural history, correlates, and treatment of major depressive disorder (MDD) in the school-aged child (6–12 years old). Although childhood depression has come under increasing scrutiny in the past decade with improved epidemiological descriptions of the phenomena, it remains a nascent discipline and outcome and treatment data are limited.

Epidemiology

Studies of school-aged children have reported prevalence rates of MDD between 0.4 per cent and 2.5 per cent with a sharp increase in its prevalence after puberty to rates similarly to those found in adults (see review by Birmaher et al., 1996). The MDD occurs approximately at the same rate in girls and boys but, again after puberty, the ratio increases to the adult proportions of approximately two females to one male (Fleming and Offord, 1990; Kessler et al., 1994; Lewinsohn et al., 1994). This sex difference has been attributed to genetics, biological changes associated with puberty, increased rates of anxiety in females, cognitive predisposition, and sociocultural factors (Reinherz et al., 1989; Rutter, 1976; Garber et al., 1994; Breslau et al., 1995; Angold et al., 1999; see also a review by Hankin and Abramson, 1999). It appears that individuals born in the latter part of the twentieth century are at greater risk for school-aged onset MDD than children born in the first half (Burke et al., 1991; Ryan et al., 1992a; Lewinsohn et al., 1993; Kovacs and Gatsonis, 1994). Thus, the prevalence has been increasing in this age group highlighting the need for further studies of MDD in school-age children.

Clinical characteristics

Depressed prepubertal children usually have depressed or irritable mood, anhedonia, changes in appetite and sleep patterns, psychomotor retardation or agitation, feelings of worthlessness, and diminished concentration. These symptoms are similar to the clinical characteristics of MDD in other age groups but there are some developmental differences. For example, instead of objectively appearing depressed, children are irritable; instead of complaining about sadness, they may endorse boredom. Children usually have more symptoms of separation anxiety, phobias, somatic complains, and behavioural problems than post-pubertal adolescents. Despite having a general sense of anhedonia their mood is more reactive and can improve with positive experiences. They rarely have the severe melancholic symptomatology often seen in adult depressed patients. Their cognitive development is reflected in suicidal plans which are not well elaborated or unrealistic (e.g. committing suicide holding their breath). When psychotic, the school-aged child usually has hallucinations (principally auditory) instead of delusions (Ryan *et al.*, 1987; Carlson and Kashani, 1988; Mitchell *et al.*, 1988; Kolvin *et al.*, 1991; Ulloa *et al.*, 2000*a*,*b*).

Several clinical and epidemiological studies have shown that the presence of comorbid psychiatric disorders is more the rule than the exception. In fact, 40–70 per cent of children with MDD have one and 20–50 per cent two or more comorbid disorders (Costello *et al.*, 1999; see also a review by Birmaher *et al.*, 1996). The most frequent comorbid diagnoses are dysthymic and anxiety disorders (both at 30–80 per cent), followed by disruptive disorders (10–80 per cent), and for older children and adolescents, substance abuse (20–30 per cent). In school-aged children MDD is more likely to occur after the onset of these comorbid psychiatric disorders; however, substance abuse usually appears in adolescents during or after an episode of depression (Kovacs *et al.*, 1989; Reinherz *et al.*, 1993; Biederman *et al.*, 1995). Behaviour problems in school aged children with MDD may develop as a complication of the depression and persist after depression remits (Kovacs *et al.*, 1988). Dysthymia usually appears to have a 2–3 year earlier onset than the first episode of MDD creating a window of opportunity for early intervention (Lewinsohn *et al.*, 1991; Kovacs *et al.*, 1994*b*).

Etiology

Genetic, psychological, and environmental factors appear to play important roles as risk factors for the occurrence and timing of onset of MDD.

Familial aggregation, twin, and adoption studies have provided evidence for genetic influences in the transmission of mood disorders (McGuffin and Murray, 1991; Reiss *et al.*, 1991; Kendler *et al.*, 1994). Studies of the offspring of depressed parents ('top-down') and of the relatives of children with MDD ('bottom-up') have shown that MDD runs in families. Lifetime risk for MDD in children of depressed parents ranges from 15 to 40 per cent (Orvaschel *et al.*, 1988; Hammen *et al.*, 1990*a*). The offspring of parents with early onset and recurrent forms of MDD, in particular if both parents are depressed, are at greatest risk for mood disorders (Weissman *et al.*, 1984, 1987, 1988; Merikangas *et al.*, 1988; Orvaschel, 1990; Mufson *et al.*, 1992). Relatives of depressed children have a 5-fold greater risk of any psychiatric illness and 2-fold greater risk of unipolar depression than psychiatric and normal controls (Kovacs *et al.*, 1997). This risk is significantly greater than the risk of the relatives of subjects with adult onset MDD indicating that childhood-onset MDD is a more familial. In the pre-pubertal child whilst familial aggregation of depression is clearly substantive there appears to be somewhat less evidence for genetic effects than in post-pubertal onset cases (Rice *et al.*, 2001). In these early years this highlights the importance of searching for non-genetic, as well as genetic, markers and precursors of depressive disorders.

So far no definitive genetic or biological markers have been found. Examination of growth hormone (GH), prolactin (PRL), and cortisol levels after pharmacological stimulation have shown abnormalities in the secretion of these hormones (e.g. blunted GH secretion after the administration of Growth Hormone Releasing Hormone; PRL and cortisol after the administration of 5-hydroxytryptophan) (see review by Birmaher and Heydl in press Boris is this now published?) Identical results have been found in never-depressed children at high risk to develop MDD due to high family loading for MDD suggesting that alteration in certain hormonal systems may be trait markers for MDD. These findings are similar to the ones found in depressed adults but other biological studies in pre-pubertal depressed subjects (e.g. the hypothalamic pituitary axis, sleep electroencephalogram) have yielded more inconsistent results with youth with melancholic symptoms, severe depressions, and older age showing same abnormalities that those reported in adults with MDD.

Twin- and adoption studies have indicated that the genetic factors account only for 50 per cent of the variance in post-pubertal cases and perhaps even less in pre-puberal (McGuffin and Murray, 1991; Kendler *et al.*, 1994; Rice *et al.*, 2001). This suggests that other factors are needed for the onset of MDD such as exposure to negative events; abuse, ongoing family conflict, and major losses have all been associated with the onset of MDD (Garber and Hilsman, 1992; Birmaher *et al.*, 1996; Williamson *et al.*, 1998; Stein *et al.*, 2000). In addition, cognitive distortions, low self-esteem, high self-criticism, and negative life view have also been associated with pre-disposition to develop depression (Jaenicke *et al.*, 1987; Hammen, 1988; Garber and Hilsman, 1992; Nolen-Hoeksema *et al.*, 1992). Current opinion suggests that biological, environmental, and psychological mechanisms interact to produce MDD (Rutter, 1990; Garber and Hilsman, 1992; Goodyer *et al.*, 1998, 2000). Thus, school-aged children who are genetically pre-disposed to develop MDD, who are exposed to an acute or ongoing stressful environments, and who have negative ways of interpreting and coping with stress are at high risk to develop depressive symptoms. Children may also have a genetic predisposition to have negative cognitions or a temperament that increases the likelihood to experience stressful events (e.g. impulsivity). Children may also learn patterns of handling stress from depressed parents that predispose them to respond with symptoms of depression (see reviews by Garber and Hilsman, 1992; Birmaher *et al.*, 1996).

Course

The average duration of a depressive episode in clinically and epidemiological samples of children is between 8 and 13 months (Kovacs *et al.*, 1984*a,b*; Goodyer *et al.*, 1997). At follow-up (12–78 months), 50–90 per cent of children with MDD recover from their depressions. However, 30–70 per cent will experience a relapse or recurrence, 24–70 months after recovery from the index episode (Poznanski *et al.*, 1976; Kovacs *et al.*, 1984*a,b*; Asarnow and Bates, 1988; McGee and Williams, 1988; McCauley *et al.*, 1993; Goodyer *et al.*, 1997; Emslie *et al.*, 1998).

It is clear that depressed school-age children are at risk to continue to experience MDD episodes during their adolescent years (see review by Birmaher *et al.* in press). However, it is not clear whether childhood onset MDD is continuous with adult MDD. Three clinical retrospective catch-up longitudinal studies that evaluated adults who were depressed during their childhood or adolescent years showed that depressed adolescents are at high risk for depression while adults but there are contradictory findings with respect the adult course of school-aged onset MDD (Harrington *et al.*, 1990; Weissman *et al.*, 2000; Fombonne *et al.*, 2001). Interestingly, childhood onset MDD was continuous with adult MDD only in children with first-degree relatives with recurrent MDD (Weissman *et al.*, 2000).

Across all studies noted above, the presence of comorbid disorders at intake predicted the persistence of these disorders during adolescence and adulthood and predicted poor academic, work, family and social functioning. Similar results have been found in adolescent-onset MDD (see review by Birmaher *et al.*, in press). Similarly to studies in depressed adolescents (Strober and Carlson *et al.*, 1982), depressed children are also at risk to develop bipolar disorder. Approximately 20–30 per cent of youth with MDD may develop bipolar disorder and require alternative psychopharmacological treatments. Children at greatest risk seem to be those with psychotic symptoms, psychomotor retardation, or pharmacologically induced hypomania (Geller *et al.*, 1994).

Some variables have consistently shown strong predictive power for recurrence of MDD including the family history for MDD (particularly of recurrent and early onset forms), the child's prior history of depression, comorbid dysthymia or anxiety disorders, and the presence of subsyndromal symptoms of depression. On the other hand, perhaps due to methodological differences, several of the risk factors including age, sex, the presence of comorbid disorders, stressful life events, and family conflicts have either not been replicated or have yielded inconsistent results. For example, some studies have found that school-aged onset is associated with the greatest hazard of recurrence (Kovacs *et al.*, 1984*a*), while others have found that adolescent onset has a greater risk of recurrence (Harrington *et al.*, 1990; Lewinsohn *et al.*, 1999). Studies addressing comorbid disruptive disorders have predicted less frequent (Harrington *et al.*, 1991), similar (Fombonne *et al.*, 2001), or more frequent recurrence of MDD (Sanford *et al.*, 1995).

Moreover, it is not clear whether some risk factors precede, appear during, or are a consequence of the MDD. In any case, even non-specific correlates are important for the management of the child's mood disorder (Garber and Hilsman, 1992). For example, ongoing family conflict is associated with more protracted episodes of depression (Asarnow *et al.*, 1994) and treatment of the conflicts may help to ameliorate, decrease episode duration, or prevent recurrence of depression in this critical developmental stage.

Few studies have investigated the biological markers associated with increased likelihood of recurrence. For example, higher cortisol/dehydroepiandrosterone (DHEA) ratio, together with one or more disappointing life events predicted persistent MDD at nine months of follow-up (Goodyer *et al.*, 1998, 2001). In addition, the onset of MDD in never-depressed adolescents was predicted by the additive effects of high salivary cortisol and DHEA level, higher depressive symptoms at intake, and personal disappointments and losses one month before onset (Goodyer *et al.*, 2001). Whether such a psycho-endocrine process is operating in the high risk pre-pubertal child prior to the onset of first episode major depression is not known. These studies emphasize the importance of simultaneously assessing clinical, environmental and biological factors, and examining their combined importance for developing MDD.

Outcome

Children with MDD have significant impairments in their school performance, perturbations of normal development, behavior problems, and relationships with parents, siblings, friends, and teachers (Rutter *et al.*, 1976; Kaslow *et al.*, 1984; Puig-Antich *et al.*, 1985*a,b*; Asarnow *et al.*, 1987, 1990; Asarnow and Ben-Meir, 1988; Hammen, 1990*a*; Kovacs and Goldston, 1991). Consequently, the developmental missteps which occur during childhood depression may have lasting effects through adolescence and adulthood.

Childhood-onset MDD leads to increased risk of tobacco use and abuse of alcohol and other substances during later adolescence (Deykin *et al.*, 1987, 1992). The fact that MDD can precede alcohol or substance abuse by an average of 4.5 years (Deykin *et al.*, 1992) again highlights the importance of treatment of depression as a pathway to preventing other forms of illness. Suicidality is also highly associated with childhood depression but at much lower rates than among adolescents (e.g. Shaffer and Fisher, 1981; Garrison *et al.*, 1991; Rao *et al.*, 1993; Brent *et al.*, 1999). Among patients who have already had one suicidal behaviour, the history of childhood depression increases risk of subsequent suicidal behaviour 7-fold compared with attempters without major depression (Pfeffer *et al.*, 1991, 1993).

Prominent psychosocial dysfunction in children with depression is marked and stands out when compared against both nonpsychiatric children as well as children without affective illness (Puig-Antich *et al.*, 1985*a*; Nolen-Koeksema *et al.*, 1992). Although the psychosocial functioning improves after remission, some impairment persist (Puig-Antich *et al.*, 1985*b*). For example, the child may continue to have subclinical symptoms of depression, negative attributions, and impairment in interpersonal relationships (Kovacs *et al.*, 1984*a,b*, 1994*b*; Puig-Antich *et al.*, 1985*b*; Nolen-Hoeksema *et al.*, 1992). Importantly, these difficulties can be accounted by the past depressive episode but to non-mood comorbid disorders or other environmental problems. All these factors may increase the risk of recurrence indicating the need of intense treatment to obtain full remission of the depressive and non-mood psychiatric symptomatology.

Treatment

There are many approaches to treatment of children with depression. It is critically important to use an approach that takes into account the family and systems issues. Family structure plays a role in etiology and prognosis of illness as discussed above. Further, children are entirely dependent upon the parents or guardians to enable access to treatment. As such, assessment and psychoeducational work with families is a critical first step in the treatment of childhood major depression (Brent *et al.*, 1993). Studies of adolescents have indicated that parents of depressed children are at increased risk for psychopathology themselves (Klein *et al.*, 2001); other studies of adolescents indicate that parental depression may lead to poor treatment response in the adolescent (Brent *et al.*, 1998). While these studies do not directly address issues of childhood depression it seems clinically prudent to carry these lessons over to the management of children and proactively assess and manage any parental issues.

Most of the randomized clinical trials of psychotherapy which included school aged children compared types of CBT or relaxation-type exercises. No studies have compared psychotherapy of any type with pharmacotherapy. There are considerable limitations in these studies including selection bias (some recruited patients seeking treatment, others recruited from screenings of school children), poor documentation of randomization, and limited outcome measures. Nonetheless the data does suggest that CBT is better than non-treatment for the management of school aged onset MDD (Votsanis *et al.*, 1996; Wood *et al.*, 1996; and see also reviews by Harrington *et al.*, 1998a,b). Interpersonal psychotherapy (IPT) has not been studied in children but is effective in adolescents (Mufson *et al.*, 1999). Family therapy—a seemingly obvious candidate for study for children—seems to have some benefit for adolescents but has not been rigorously studied in school age children (Harrington, 1998a).

More severe and chronic depressions, those with significant comorbid disorders, with parental conflict and psychopathology often fail respond to monotherapy with psychotherapy or pharmacotherapy alone (Emslie *et al.*, 1998). Therefore, severe and chronic depressions should be treated with both antidepressants and psychotherapy. Other risk factors for poor outcome (e.g. parent depression, child ADHD), should be addressed with additional psychosocial and pharmacological interventions as necessary.

Tricyclic antidepressants have been studied as a treatment for childhood depression. With the exception of Preskorn *et al.* (1987), who found a statistically significant but clinically small antidepressant effect in one of the outcome measurements, all of the controlled double-blind trials have reported no significant differences between placebo and TCAs (Petti and Law, 1982; Kashani *et al.*, 1984; Puig-Antich *et al.*, 1987; Geller *et al.*, 1989; Hughes *et al.*, 1990). While the number of TCA studies in children is quite small compared with the number of studies in adults (e.g. Burke and

Preskorn, 1995) the lackluster results do not tend to inspire one to study them further. Moreover, TCAs also do not seem to be useful for the treatment of depressed adolescents (Birmaher *et al.*, 1996; Keller *et al.*, 2001). One reason for the poor response of childhood vs adult MDD to TCAs is that most of the child studies used tertiary amines or noradrenergic TCAs resulting in some greater noradrenergic effects. The noradrenergic system is not fully developed until early adulthood (e.g. Murrin *et al.*, 1985; Nordberg, 1986). Some phenomenological characteristics of childhood depression may also help us to understand children's response to medications. For example, more children and adolescents show transition into bipolar disorder than adults (Strober and Carlson, 1982; Geller *et al.*, 1994), and in adults, bipolar depression seems to be less responsive to TCAs (Himmelhoch *et al.*, 1991). Finally, children have more efficient hepatic metabolism of drugs than adults resulting in rapid deamination of TCAs, and, as a consequence relatively less serotonergic amine TCAs available (Clein and Riddle, 1995; Kye and Ryan, 1995); this will again become important in the discussion of SSRIs.

The reports that SSRIs are efficacious for the treatment of adults with MDD (APA, 2000) together with the findings that SSRIs are efficacious and safe for other childhood psychiatric disorders (e.g. anxiety disorders and obsessive compulsive disorder) have a relatively safe side effect profile, very low lethality in overdose, and easy administration have lead to the widespread use of SSRIs as first line treatment for MDD in children (Leonard, 1997; Emslie *et al.*, 1999). All SSRIs appear to be equally efficacious for the treatment of adult major depression and have relatively similar side effect profiles. This seems to be true for children as well as adolescents and adults however children seem to metabolize the SSRIs and other antidepressants quicker than adults and—at least at low dosages—need twice daily dosing (Clein and Riddle, 1995; Findling *et al.*, 1999; 2000; Axelson *et al.*, 2000 *a,b*).

Despite the endemic use of SSRI's for childhood depression there are relatively few studies, controlled or otherwise. In two randomized controlled trials fluoxetine was shown to be more effective than placebo in regulating childhood major depression (Emslie *et al.*, 1997*b*, 2000). Despite the significant response to fluoxetine, many patients had only partial improvement and a substantial proportion did not remitted. The low rate of response may be due to a low dose or brief duration of treatment. A follow up of the subjects who participated in the above noted an improved rate as the duration of treatment increased (Emslie *et al.*, 1998). The combination of psychotherapy with medications may have increased the number of responders in these studies.

Other antidepressants, including the heterocyclics (e.g. amoxapine, maprotiline); bupropion, venlafaxine, and nefazodone, have been found to be efficacious for the treatment of depressed adults (APA, 2000), but studies in children are rare. One study of including a very small sample of school age children with MDD found that venlafaxine was a well tolerated but clinically unimpressive treatment (Mandoki *et al.*, 1997).

As noted previously, children with MDD are at increased risk for eventual bipolarity compared with adolescents and adults; a prospective study of high-risk children (family history of bipolar disorder) treated with lithium revealed no difference in outcome compared with placebo (Geller *et al.*, 1998). A few open studies have also shown that MAOIs can be used safely with children and adolescents (Ryan *et al.*, 1988), but noncompliance with dietary requirements may present a significant problem for youth. Electroconvulsive therapy is used rarely in children and has not been studied systematically; one of two published cases where ECT was chosen for childhood catatonic MDD had a positive outcome (Cizaldo and Wheaton, 1995; Fink and Carlson, 1995). There has been one randomized, controlled trial of light therapy which showed positive results for a mixed population of twenty eight children aged 7–17 years however specific subgroup data on the younger children is not provided (Swedo *et al.*, 1997).

Naturalistic studies in children indicate that continuation of pharmacotherapy can decrease the rates of recurrence (Emslie *et al.*, 1998). Similar studies in adults and adolescents have found similar effects for both pharmacotherapy and psychotherapy (Fava *et al.*, 1996; Kroll *et al.*, 1996; Mufson and Fairbanks, 1996). Thus, although not well studied in children, it seems clinically reasonable to continue treatment to prevent relapses and recurrences for at least 6–12 months. Patients who are maintained only on medications should continue the same medication dosage and be offered psychotherapy to help them cope with the 'psychosocial scars' induced by the depression. Furthermore, many depressed youth have non-mood comorbid psychiatric disorders and they live in environments charged with stressful situations and their parents usually have psychiatric disorders, emphasizing the need for multimodal treatments. The reduction of family stress, promotion of a supportive environment, and effective treatment of parents and siblings with psychiatric disorders may also help diminish the risk for recurrence (Stein *et al.*, 2000).

Children, who have shown difficulty achieving remission from depression, have had two or more recurrent episodes of MDD, psychosis, or significant suicidality should be offered maintenance treatment to avoid recurrences for one year or more. Other factors which would suggest use of a longer initial treatment course include persistent subsyndromal symptoms of depression, early onset, family history of recurrent depression, dysthymia, comorbid disorders, and ongoing exposure to stressors such as family discord (Birmaher *et al.*, 1996; AACAP, 1998).

Conclusion

School-aged depression is a familial, identifiable, and treatable phenomena which often occurs in complex family environments and with multiple comorbid disorders. Childhood-onset MDD is associated with increased risks of later psychopathology including unipolar and bipolar depression, substance use, and psychosocial problems. This highlights the importance of prevention, early identification, adequate treatment and follow-up of childhood depression.

While few psychosocial and pharmacological studies have shown their efficacy and safety for the acute treatment of school-age children with MDD, more acute and long term blinded, randomized trials are needed in order to fine tune treatment strategies with an emphasis on prevention of recurrences and long term safety of the new antidepressants.

Childhood depression is associated with multiple comorbidities and often-complex psychosocial environments. While this makes treatment and outcome studies difficult, these remain critically important fields for future study.

References

American Academy of Children and Adolescent Psychiatry (AACAP) (1998). Practice parameters for the assessment and treatment of children and adolescents with depressive disorder. *Journal of the American Academy of Child and Adolescent Psychiatry*, **37**(Supplement), 63S–83S.

American Psychiatric Association (APA) (2000). Practice for the treatment of patients with major depressive disorder (revision). *American Journal of Psychiatry*, **157**(Supplement), 1–45.

Angold, A., Costello, E.J., and Erkanli, A. (1999). Comorbidity. *Journal of Child Psychology, Psychiatry, and Allied Disciplines*, **40**, 57–87.

Asarnow, J.R., Tompson, M., Hamilton, E.B., Goldstein, M.J. *et al.* (1994). Family expressed emotion, childhood-onset depression, and childhood-onset schizophrenia spectrum disorders: Is expressed emotion a nonspecific correlate of child psychopathology or a specific risk factor for depression? *Journal of Abnormal Child Psychology*, **22**, 129–146.

Asarnow, J.R. and Ben-Meir, S. (1988). Children with schizophrenia spectrum and depressive disorders: a comparative study of premorbid adjustment, onset pattern and severity of impairment. *Journal of Child Psychology and Psychiatry*, **29**, 477–488.

Asarnow, J.R. and Bates, S. (1988). Depression in child psychiatric inpatients: cognitive and attributional patterns. *Journal of Abnormal Child Psychology*, **16**, 601–615.

Asarnow, J.R., Carlson, G., and Guthrie, D. (1987). Coping strategies, self-perceptions, hopelessness, and perceived family environments in depressed and suicidal children. *Journal of Consulting and Clinical Psychology*, **55**, 361–366.

Asarnow, J.R., Goldstein, M., Marshall, V., and Weber, E. (1990). Mother-child dynamics in early onset depression and childhood schizophrenia spectrum disorders. *Developmental Psychopathology*, **2**, 71–84.

Axelson, D., Perel, J., Rudolph, G., Birmaher, B., and Brent, D. (2000a). Sertraline pediatric/adolescent PK-PD parameters: Dose/plasma level ranging for depression (Abstract). *Clinical Pharmacology and Therapeutics*, **67**, 169.

Axelson, D., Perel, J., Rudolph, G., Birmaher, B., Nuss, S., and Brent, D. (2000b). Significant differences in pharmacokinetics/dynamics of ±Citalopram between adolescents and adults: Implications for clinical dosing [Abstract]. *Proceedings of the 39th Annual Meeting of the American College of Neuropsychopharmacology* San Juan, Puerto Rico, (pp. 122).

Biederman, J., Faraone, S., Mick, E., and Lelon, E. (1995). Psychiatric comorbidity among referred juveniles with major depression: fact or artifact? *Journal of the American Academy of Child and Adolescent Psychiatry*, **34**, 579–590.

Birmaher, B. and Heydl, P. (2001). Biological studies in depressed children and adolescents. *International Journal of Neuropsychopharmacology*, **4**, 149–157.

Birmaher, B., Arbelaez, C., and Brent, D. (2002). Course and outcome of child and adolescent major depressive disorder. *Child and Adolescent Psychiatric Clinics of North America*, **11**, 619–638.

Birmaher, B., Ryan, N.D., Williamson, D., Brent, D., Kaufman, J., Dahl, R., Perel, J., and Nelson, B. (1996). Childhood and adolescent depression: A review of the past 10 years—Part I. *Journal of the American Academy of Child and Adolescent Psychiatry*, **35**, 1427–1439.

Brent, D.A., Perper, J.A., Goldstein, C.E., Kolko, D.J., Allan, M., Allman, C.J., and Zelenak, J.P. (1988). Risk factor for adolescent suicide: a comparison of adolescent suicide victims with suicidal inpatients. *Archives of General Psychiatry*, **45**, 581–588.

Brent, D.A., Poling, K., McKain B., and Baugher, M. (1993). A Psychoeducational program for families of affectively ill children and adolescents. *Journal of the American Academy of Child and Adolescent Psychiatry*, **32**, 770–774.

Brent, D.A., Kolko, D., Birmaher, B., Baugher, M., Bridge, J., Roth, C., and Holder, D. (1998). Predictors of treatment efficacy in a clinical trial of three psychosocial treatments for adolescent depression. *Journal of the American Academy of Child and Adolescent Psychiatry*, **37**, 906–914.

Brent, D.A., Baugher M., Bridge J., Chen J., and Beery L. (1999). Age and sex-related risk factors for adolescent suicide. *Journal of the American Academy of Child and Adolescent Psychiatry*, **38**, 1497–1505.

Breslau, N., Schultz, L., and Peterson E. (1995). Sex differences in depression: a role for preexisting anxiety. *Psychiatry Research*, **58**, 1–12.

Burke, K.C., Burke, J.D., Rae, D.S., and Regier, D.A. (1991). Comparing age at onset of major depression and other psychiatric disorders by birth cohorts in five US community populations. *Archives of General Psychiatry*, **48**, 789–795.

Burke, M.J. and Preskorn, S.H. (1995). Short-term treatment of mood disorders with standard antidepressants. In: *Psychopharmacology: The Fourth Generation of Progress* Bloom, F.E. and Kupfer, D.J. (Eds.), Raven Press, New York, pp. 1053–1065.

Carlson, G.A. and Kashani, J.H. (1988). Phenomenology of major depression from childhood through adulthood: analysis of three studies. *American Journal of Psychiatry*, **30**, 144–150.

Cizaldo, B.C. and Wheaton, A. (1995). Case Study: ECT Treatment of a young girl with catatonia. *Journal of the American Academy of Child and Adolescent Psychiatry*, **34**, 332–335.

Clein, P.D. and Riddle, M.A. (1995). Pharmacokinetics in children and adolescents. *Child and Adolescent Psychiatric Clinics of North America*, **4**, 59–75.

Costello, E.J., Erkanli, A., Federman, E., and Angold, A. (1999). Development of psychiatric comorbidity with substance abuse in adolescents: Effects of timing and sex. *Journal of Clinical Child Psychology*, **28**, 298–311.

Deykin, E.Y., Buka, S.L., and Zeena, T.H. (1992). Depressive illness among chemically dependent adolescents. *American Journal of Psychiatry*, **149**, 1341–1347.

Deykin, E.Y., Levy, J.C., and Wells, V. (1987). Adolescent depression, alcohol and drug abuse. *American Journal of Public Health*, **77**, 178–182.

Emslie, G.J., Walkup, J.T., Pliszka, S.R., and Ernst, M. (1999). Nontricyclic antidepressants: Current trends in children and adolescents. *Journal of the American Academy for Child and Adolescent Psychiatry*, **38**, 517–528.

Emslie, G., Rush, A.J., Weinberg, A.W., Kowatch, R.A., Hughes, C.W., Carmody, T., and Rintelmann, J. (1997*b*). A double-blind, randomized placebo-controlled trial of fluoxetine in depressed children and adolescents. *Archives of General Psychiatry*, **54**, 1031–1037.

Emslie, G.J., Heiligenstein, J.H., Hoog, S.L., Judge, R., Brown, E.B., and Nilsson, M. (2000). Fluoxetine for acute treatment of depression in children and adolescents: A placebo controlled randomized clinical trial. Presented at the 39th Annual Meeting of the American College of Neuropsychopharmacology. San Juan, Puerto Rico.

Emslie, G.J., Rush, A.J., Weinberg, W.A., Gullion, C.M., Rintelmann, J., and Hughes, C.W. (1997*a*). Recurrence of major depressive disorder in hospitalized children and adolescents. *Journal of the American Academy of Child and Adolescent Psychiatry*, **36**, 785–792.

Emslie, G.J., Rush, A.J., Weinberg, W.A., Kowatch, R.A., Carmody, T., and Mayes, T.L. (1998). Fluoxetine in child and adolescent depression: Acute and maintenance treatment. *Depress. Anxiety*, **7**, 32–39.

Fava, G.A., Grandi, S., Zielezny, M., Rafanelli, C., and Caneatrari, R. (1996). Four-year outcome for cognitive behavioral treatment of residual symptoms in major depression. *American Journal of Psychiatry*, **153**, 945–947.

Fendrich, M., Warner, V., and Weissman, M. (1990). Family risk factors, parental depression, and childhood psychopathology. *Developmental Psychology*, **26**, 40–50.

Findling, R.L., Reed, M.D., Myers, C., Riordan, M.A., Fiala, S., Branicky, L., Waldorf, B., and Blumer, J.L. (1999). Paroxetine pharmacokinetics in depressed children and adolescents. *Journal of the American Academy of Child and Adolescent Psychiatry*, **38**, 952–959.

Findling, R.L., Preskorn, S.H., Marcus, R.N., Magnus, R.D., D'Amico, F., Marathe, P., and Reed, M.D. (2000). Nefazodone pharmacokinetics in depressed children and adolescents. *Journal of the American Academy of Child and Adolescent Psychiatry*, **39**, 1008–1016.

Fink, M. and Carlson, G.A. (1995). ECT and prepubertal children [Correspondence]. *Journal of the American Academy of Child and Adolescent Psychiatry*, **34**, 1256–1257.

Fleming, J.E. and Offord, D.R. (1990). Epidemiology of childhood depressive disorders: a critical review. *Journal of the American Academy of Child and Adolescent Psychiatry*, **29**, 571–580.

Fombonne, E., Wostear, G., Cooper, V. *et al.* (2001). The Maudsley long term follows up of child and adolescent depression. Psychiatric outcomes in adulthood. *British Journal of Psychiatry*, **179**, 210–217.

Garber, J. and Hilsman, R. (1992), Cognition, stress, and depression in children and adolescents, *Child and Adolescent Psychiatric Clinics of North America*.

Garber, J., Robinson, N.S., Little, S., and Hilsman, R. (1994). Stress and depression: Risk and protective factors in girls versus boys. Presented at the American Academy of Child and Adolescent Psychiatry Meeting, New York.

Garrison, C.Z., Jackson, K.L., Addy, C.L., McKeown, R.E., and Waller, J.L. (1991), Suicidal behaviors in young adolescents. *American Journal of Epidemiology*, **133**, 1005–1014.

Geller, B., Cooper, T., McCombs, H., Graham, D., and Wells, J. (1989). Double-blind, placebo-controlled study of nortriptyline in depressed children using a 'fixed plasma level' design. *Psychopharmacology Bulletin*, **25**, 101–108.

Geller, B., Fox, L.W., and Clark, K.A. (1994). Rate and predictors of prepubertal bipolarity during follow-up of 6- to 12-year-old depressed children. *Journal of the American Academy of Child and Adolescent Psychiatry*, **33**, 461–468.

Geller, B., Cooper, T., Zimerman, B., Frazier, J., Williams, M., Heath, J., and Warner, K. (1998). Lithium for prepubertal depressed children with family history predictors of future bipolarity: a double-blind, placebo-controlled study. *Journal of affective Disorders*, **51**, 165–175.

Goodyer, I.M., Herbert, J., Secher, S.M., and Pearson, J. (1997). Short-term outcome of major depression: I. Comorbidity and severity at presentation as predictors of persistent disorder. *Journal of the American Academy of Child and Adolescent Psychiatry*, **36**, 179–187.

Goodyer, I.M., Herbert, J., and Altham, P.M.E. (1998). Adrenal steroid secretion and major depression in 8- to 16-yr-olds: III. Influence of cortisol/DHEA ratio at presentation on subsequent rates of disappointing life events and persistent major depression. *Psychological Medicine*, **28**, 265–273.

Goodyer, I.M., Park, R.J., and Herbert, J. (2001). Psychosocial and endocrine features of chronic first-episode major depression in 8–16 year olds. *Biological Psychiatry*, **50**, 351–357.

Goodyer, I.M., Herbert, J., Tamplin, A., and Altham, P.M.E. (2000). Recent life events, cortisol, dehydroepiandrosterone and the onset of major depression in high-risk adolescents. *British Journal of Psychiatry*, **177**, 499–504.

Hammen, C. (1988). Self-cognition, stressful events, and the prediction of depression in children of depressed mother. *Journal of Abnormal Child Psychology*, **16**, 347–360.

Hammen, C., Burge, D., Burney, E., and Adrian, C. (1990a). Longitudinal study of diagnoses in children of women with unipolar and bipolar affective disorder. *Archives of General Psychiatry*, **47**, 1112–1117.

Hammen, C., Burge, D., and Stanbury, K. (1990b). Relationship of mother and child variables to child outcomes in a high-risk sample: a casual modeling analysis. *Developmental Psychology*, **26**, 24–30.

Hankin, B.L. and Abramson, L.Y. (1999). Development of gender differences in depression: description and possible explanations. *Annals of Medicine*, **31**, 372–379.

Harrington, R., Fudge, H., Rutter, M., Pickles, A., and Hill, J. (1990). Adult outcomes of child and adolescent depression: I. Psychiatric status. *Archives of General Psychiatry*, **47**, 465–473.

Harrington, R., Fudge, H., Rutter, M., Pickles, A. *et al.* (1991). Adult outcomes of child and adolescent depression: II. Links with antisocial disorders. *Archives of General Psychiatry*, **47**, 465–473.

Harrington, R., Whittaker, J., and Shoebridge, P. (1998a). Psychological treatment of depression in children and adolescents. A review of treatment research. *British Journal of Psychiatry*, **173**, 291–298.

Harrington, R., Whittaker, J., Shoebridge, P., and Campbell, F. (1998b). Systematic review of efficacy of cognitive behaviour therapies in childhood and adolescent depressive disorder. *British Medical Journal*, **316**, 1559–1563.

Himmelhoch, J., Thase, M., Mallinger, A., and Houck, P. (1991). Tranylcypromine versus imipramine in anergic bipolar depression. *American Journal of Psychiatry*, **148**, 910–916.

Hughes, C.W., Preskorn, S., Weller, E., Weller, R., Hassanein, R., and Tucker, S. (1990). The effect of concomitant disorders in childhood depression on predicting treatment response. *Psychopharmacology Bullein*, **26**, 235–238.

Jaenicke, C., Hammen, C., Zupan, B., *et al.* (1987). Cognitive vulnerability in children at risk for depression. *Journal of Abnormal Child Psychology*, **15**, 1559–572.

Kashani, J., Shekim, W., and Reid, J. (1984). Amitriptyline in children with major depressive disorder: A double-blind crossover pilot study. *Journal of the American Academy of Child and Adolescent Psychiatry*, 23, 348–351.

Kaslow, N., Rehm, L., and Siegel, A. (1984). Social-cognitive and cognitive correlates of depression in children. *Journal of Abnormal Child Psychology*, 12, 605–620.

Keller, M.B., Ryan, N.D., Strober, M.K., *et al.* (2001) Efficacy of paroxetine in the treatment of adolescent major depression: A randomized, controlled trial. *Journal of the American Academy of Child & Adolescent Psychiatry*, 40, 762–772.

Kendler, K.S., Walters, E.E., Truett, K.R., Keath, A.C., Neale, M.C., Martin, N.G., and Eaves, L.J. (1994). Sources of individual differences in depressive symptoms: analysis of two samples of twins and their families. *American Journal of Psychiatry*, 151, 1605–1614.

Kessler, R.C., McGonagle, K.A., Nelson, C.B., Hughes, M., Swartz, M., and Blazer, D.G. (1994). Sex and depression in the national comorbidity survey: II. Cohort effects. *Journal of Affective Disorders*, 30, 15–26.

Klein, D.N., Lewinsohn, P.M., Seeley, J.R., and Rohde, P. (2001). A family study of major depressive disorder in a community sample of adolescents. *Archives of General Psychiatry*, 58, 13–20.

Kolvin, I., Barrett, M.L., Berney, T.P., Famuyiwa, O.O., Fundudis, T., and Tryer, S. (1991). The Newcastle child depression project; Diagnosis and classification of depression. *British Journal of Psychiatry*, 159, 28–25.

Kovacs, M., Feinberg, T.L., Crouse-Novak, M.A., Paulauskas, S.L., and Finkelstein, R. (1984*a*). Depressive disorders in childhood: I. A longitudinal prospective study of characteristics and recovery. *Archives of General Psychiatry*, 41, 229–237.

Kovacs, M., Feinberg, T.L., Crouse-Novak, M., Paulaskas, S.L., and Pollock, M., and Finkelstein, R. (1984*b*). Depressive disorders in childhood. II. A longitudinal study of the risk for a subsequent major depression. *Archives of General Psychiatry*, 41, 643–649.

Kovacs, M., Gatsonis, C., Paulauskas, S., and Richards, C. (1989). Depressive disorders in childhood: IV. A longitudinal study of comorbidity with and risk for anxiety disorders. *Archives of General Psychiatry*, 46, 776–782.

Kovacs, M. and Goldston, D. (1991). Cognitive and social cognitive development of depressed children and adolescents. *Journal of the American Academy of Child and Adolescent Psychiatry*, 30, 388–392.

Kovacs, M., Gatsonis, C. (1994*a*). Secular trends in age at onset of major depressive disorder in a clinical sample of children. *Journal of Psychiatry Research*, 28, 319–329.

Kovacs, M., Akiskal, S., Gatsonis, C., and Parrone, P.L. (1994*b*). Childhood-onset dysthymic disorder. *Archives of General Psychiatry*, 51, 365–374.

Kovacs, M., Devlin, B., Pollock, M., Richards, C., and Mukerji, P. (1997). A controlled family history study of childhood-onset depressive disorder. *Archives of General Psychiatry*, 54, 613–623.

Kovacs, M., Paulauska, S., Gatsonis, C., and Richards, C. (1988). Depressive disorders in childhood III: A longitudinal study of comorbidity and risk for conduct disorders. *Journal of Affective Disorders*, 15, 205–217.

Kroll, L., Harrington, R., Jayson, D., Fraser, J., and Gowers, S. (1996). Pilot study of continuation cognitive-behavioral therapy for major depression in adolescent psychiatric patients. *Journal of the American Academy of Child and Adolescent Psychiatry*, 35, 1156–1161.

Kye, C. and Ryan, N.D. (1995). Pharmacologic treatment of child and adolescent depression. *Child and Adolescent Psychiatric Clinics of North America*, 4, 261–281.

Leonard, H.L., March, J., Rickler, K.C., and Allen, A.J. (1997). Review of the pharmacology of the selective serotonin reuptake inhibitors in children and adolescents. *Journal of the American Academy of Child and Adolescent Psychiatry*, 36, 725–736.

Lewinsohn, P.M., Clarke, G.N., Seeley, J.R., and Rohde, P. (1994). Major depression in community adolescents: age at onset, episode duration, and time to recurrence. *Journal of the American Academy of Child and Adolescent Psychiatry*, 33(6), 809–818.

Lewinsohn, P.M., Allen, N.B., Seeley, J.R., and Gotlib, I.H. (1999). First onset versus recurrence of depression: Differential processes of psychosocial risk. *Journal of Abnormal Psychology*, 108, 483–489.

Lewinsohn, P.M., Rohde, P., Seeley, J.R., and Fischer, S.A. (1993). Age-cohort changes in the lifetime occurrence of depression and other mental disorders. *Journal of Abnormal Psychology*, 102, 110–120.

Lewinsohn, P.M., Rohde, P., Seeley, J.R., and Hops, H. (1991). Comorbidity of unipolar depression I: Major depression with dysthymia. *Journal of Abnormal Psychology*, 100, 205–213.

Mandoki, M.W., Tapia, M.R., Tapia, M.A., and Sumner, G.S. (1997). Venlafaxine in the treatment of children and adolescents with major depression. *Psychopharmacology Bulletin*, 33, 149–154.

McCauley, E., Myers, K., Mitchel, J., Calderon, R., Schloredt, K., and Treder, R. (1993). Depression in young people: initial presentation and clinical course. *Journal of the American Academy of Child and Adolescent Psychiatry*, 32, 714–722.

McGee, R. and Williams, S. (1988). A longitudinal study of depression in nine-year-old children, *Journal of the American Academy of Child and Adolescent Psychiatry*, 27, 342–348.

McGuffin, P. and Murray, R. (1991). *The New Genetics of Mental Illness*. Oxford: Butterworth-Heinemann.

Merikangas, K.R., Weissman, M.M., Prusoff, B.A., and John, K. (1988). Assortative mating and affective disorders: psychopathology in offspring. *Psychiatry*, 51, 48–57.

Mitchell, J., McCauley, E., Burle, P.M., and Mass, S.J. (1988). Phenomenology of depression in children and adolescents. *Journal of the American Academy Child and Adolescent Psychiatry*, 12–20.

Mufson, L., Weissman, M.M., and Warner, V. (1992). Depression and anxiety in parents and children: a direct interview study. *Journal of Anxiety Disorders*, 6, 1–13.

Mufson, L. and Fairbanks, J. (1996). Interpersonal psychotherapy for depressed adolescents: A one-year naturalistic follow-up study. *Journal of the American Academy of Child and Adolescent Psychiatry*, 35, 1145–1155.

Mufson, L., Weissman, M.M., Moreau, D., and Garfinkel, R. (1999). Efficacy of interpersonal psychotherapy for depressed adolescents. *Archives of General Psychiatry*, 56, 573–579.

Murrin, L., Gibbens, D., and Ferrer, J. (1985). Ontogeny of dopamine, serotonin, and spirocecanone receptors in rat forebrain: An autoradiographic study. *Developmental Brain Research*, 23, 91–109.

Nolen-Hoeksema, S., Girgus, J.S., and Seligman, M.E.P. (1992). Predictors and consequences of childhood depressive symptoms: A 5-year longitudinal study. *Journal of Abnormal Psychology*, 101, 405–422.

Nordberg, A. (1986). The aging of cholinergic synapses: Ontogenesis of cholinergic receptors. In Dynamics of Cholinergic Function: I. Hannin (Ed.). Plenum, New York, pp. 165–175.

Orvaschel, H. (1990). Early onset psychiatric disorder in high risk children and increased family morbidity. *Journal of the American Academy of Child and Adolescent Psychiatry*, 29, 184–188.

Orvaschel, H., Walsh-Allis, G., and Ye, W. (1988). Psychopathology in children of parents with recurrent depression. *Journal of Abnormal Child Psychology*, 16, 17–28.

Petti, T. and Law, W. (1982). Imipramine treatment of depressed children: a double-blind pilot study. *Journal of Clinical Psychopharmacology*, 2, 107–110.

Pfeffer, C.R., Klerman, G.L., Hurt, S.W., Lesser, M., Peskin, J.R., and Siefker, C.A. (1991). Suicidal children grow up: demographic and clinical risk factors for adolescent suicide attempts. *Journal of the American Academy of Child and Adolescent Psychiatry*, 30, 609–616.

Pfeffer, C.R., Klerman, G.L., Hurt, S.W., Kakuma, T. *et al.* (1993). Suicidal children grow up: rates and psychosocial risk factors for suicide attempts during follow up. *Journal of the American Academy of Child and Adolescent Psychiatry*, 32, 106–113.

Poznanski, E.O., Krahenbuhl, V., and Zrull, J.P. (1976). Childhood depression: A longitudinal perspective. *Journal of the American Academy of Child Psychiatry*, 15, 491–501.

Preskorn, S.H., Weller, E.B., Hughes, C.W., Weller, R.A., and Bolte, K. (1987). Depression in prepubertal children: Dexamethasone nonsuppression predicts differential response to imipramine vs. placebo. *Psychopharmacology Bulletin*, 23, 128–133.

Puig-Antich, J., Lukens, E., Davies, M., Goetz, D., Brennan-Quattrock, J., and Todak, G. (1985a). Psychosocial functioning in prepubertal depressive disorders I: Interpersonal relationships during the episode. *Archives of General Psychiatry*, 42, 500–507.

Puig-Antich, J., Lukens, E., Davies, M., Goetz, D., Brennan-Quattrock J., and Todak, G. (1985b). Psychosocial functioning in prepubertal depressive disorders II: Interpersonal relationships after sustained recovery from affective illness. *Archives of General Psychiatry*, 42, 511–517.

Puig-Antich, J., Perel, J., Lupatkin, W., *et al.* (1987). Imipramine in prepubertal major depressive disorders. *Archives of General Psychiatry*, 44, 81–89.

Rao, U., Weissman, M.M., Martin, J.A., and Hammond, R.W. (1993). Childhood depression and risk of suicide: a preliminary report of a longitudinal study. *Journal of the American Academy of Child and Adolescent Psychiatry*, 32, 21–27.

Reinherz, H.Z., Giaconia, R.M., Pakis, B., Silverman, A.B., Frost, A.K., and Lefkowitz, E.S. (1993). Psychosocial risks for major depression in late adolescence: a longitudinal community study. *Journal of the American Academy of Child and Adolescent Psychiatry*, 32, 1155–1163.

Reinherz, H.Z., Stewart-Berghauer, G., Pakiz, B., Frost, A.K., Moeykens, B.A., and Holmes, W.M. (1989). The relationship of early risk and current mediators to depressive symptomatology in adolescence. *Journal of the American Academy of Child and Adolescent Psychiatry*, 28, 942–937.

Reiss, D., Plomin, R., and Hetherington, E.M. (1991). Genetics and psychiatry: an unheralded window on the environment. *American Journal of Psychiatry*, 148, 283–291.

Rice, F., Harold, G. *et al.* (2001). 'The genetic aetiology of childhood depression: a review'. *Journal of Child Psychology and Psychiatry*, 43(1), 65–79.

Rutter, M. (1990). Commentary: Some focus and process considerations regarding effects of parental depression on children. *Developmental Psychology*, 26, 60–67.

Rutter, M. *et al.* (1976). Isle of Wight studies 1964–1974. *Psychological Medicine*, 6, 313–332.

Ryan, N., Meyer, V., Dachille, S., Mazzie, D., and Puig-Antich, J. (1988). Lithium antidepressant augmentation in TCA-refractory depression in adolescents. *Journal of the American Academy of Child and Adolescent Psychiatry*, 27, 371–376.

Ryan, N.D., Puig-Antich, J., Ambrosini, P., Rabinovich, H., Robinson, D., Nelson, B., Iyengar, S., and Twomey, J. (1987). The clinical picture of major depression in children and adolescents. *Archives of General Psychiatry*, 44, 854–861.

Ryan, N.D., Williamson, D.E., Iyengar, S., Orvaschel, H. *et al.* (1992a). A secular increase in child and adolescent onset affective disorder. *Journal of the American Academy of Child and Adolescent Psychiatry*, 31, 600–605.

Sanford, M., Szatmari, P., Spinner, M., Munroe-Blum, H. *et al.* (1995). Predicting the one-year course of adolescent major depression. *Journal of the American Academy of Child and Adolescent Psychiatry*, 34, 1618–1628.

Shaffer, D. and Fisher, P. (1981). The epidemiology of suicide in children and young adolescents. *Journal of the American Academy of Child Psychiatry*, 20, 545–561.

Stein, D., Williamson, D.E., Birmaher, B., Brent, D.A., Kaufman, J., Dahl, R.E., and Ryan, N.D. (2000). Parent-child bonding and family functioning in depressed children and children at high-risk and low risk for future depression. *Journal of the American Academy of Child and Adolescent Psychiatry*, **39**, 1220–1226.

Strober, M. and Carlson, G. (1982). Predictors of bipolar illness in adolescents with major depression: A follow-up investigation. *Adolescent Psychiatry*, **10**, 299–319.

Swedo, S.E., Allen, A.J., Glod, C.A., *et al.* (1997). A controlled trial of light therapy for the treatment of pediatric seasonal affective disorder. *Journal of the American Academy of Child and Adolescent Psychiatry*, **36**, 816–821.

Ulloa, R.E., Apiquian, R., Fresan, A., and de la Pena, F. (2000*a*). Child and adolescent psychosis: A review of characteristics and treatment. *Salud Mental*, **23**, 1–9.

Ulloa, R.E., Birmaher, B., Axelson, D., Williamson, D.E., Brent, D.A., Ryan, N.D., Bridge, J., and Baugher, M. (2000*b*). Psychosis in a pediatric mood and anxiety disorders clinic: Phenomenology and correlates. *Journal of the American Academy of Child and Adolescent Psychiatry*, **39**, 337–345.

Vostanis, P., Feehan, C., Grattan, E., and Bickerton, W.A. (1996). A randomized controlled outpatient trial of cognitive- behavioral treatment for children and adolescents with depression: 9-month follow-up. *Journal of Affective Disorders*, **40**, 105–116.

Williamson, D.E., Birmaher, B., and Frank, E. (1998). Nature of life events and difficulties in depressed adolescents. *Journal of the American Academy of Child and Adolescent Psychiatry*, **37**, 1049–1057.

Weissman, M.M., Warner, V., Wickramaratne, P., and Prusoff, B.A. (1988). Early-onset major depression in parents and their children. *Journal of Affective Disorders*, **15**, 269–277.

Weissman, M.M., Wickramaratne, P., and Merikangas, K.R., Leckman, J.F., Prusoff, B.A., Caruso, K.A., Kidd, K.K., and Gammon, G.D. (1984). Onset of major depression in early adulthood: increase in familial loading and specificity. *Archives of General Psychiatry*, **41**, 1136–1143.

Weissman, M.M., Warner, V., Wickramaratne, P., Moreau, D., and Olfson, M. (2000). Offspring at risk: Early-onset major depresson and anxiety disorders over a decade. In J.L. Rapoport (Ed.) Childhood onset of 'adult' psychopathology: Clinical and Research Advances, American Psychopathological Association Series. American Psychiatric Press, Washington, DC, US (pp. 245–258).

Weissman, M.M., Gammon, G.D., John, K., Merikangas, K.R., Prusoff, B.A., and Sholomskas, D. (1987) Children of depressed parents: Increased psychopathology and early onset of major depression. *Archives of General Psychiatry*, **44**, 847–853.

Wood, A., Harrington, R., and Moore, A. (1996). Controlled trial of a brief cognitive-behavioral intervention in adolescent patients with depressive disorders. *Journal of Child Psychology and Psychiatry*, **37**, 737–746.

Chapter 4

Adolescence

Richard Harrington

Concepts

The concept of a depressive syndrome that is distinct from the broad class
of other adolescent emotional disorders has a relatively short history.
Until the 1970s it was believed that depressive disorders resembling adult
depression were uncommon among the young. Young adolescents were
thought incapable of experiencing depression. Depression in older adolescents was often seen as a normal feature of development, the so-called
adolescent turmoil. However, in the 1970s and early 1980s several investigators began to diagnose depression in young people using adult criteria
(Weinberg *et al.*, 1973; Pearce, 1978; Puig-Antich, 1982). These studies showed
that conditions resembling adult depression could occur from middle
childhood upwards. Indeed, recent epidemiological studies have reported
that as many as one in ten adolescent girls suffer from depressive disorders
(Olsson and von Knorring, 1999; Angold *et al.*, 1999b).

Since these estimates come from the application of operational criteria in
the Diagnostic and Statistical Manual (American Psychiatric Association,
1987, 1994), which states that the core symptoms of depression in young
people are the same as adults, it might be thought that any remaining
doubts about the validity of the concept had been dispelled. This is not the
case. There are still uncertainties.

The first concerns the distinction between depressive disorder and nor-
mality. Symptoms of depression such as sadness and sleep disturbance are
very common in adolescence. The usual way of differentiating such symptoms from depression as a disorder is to apply some kind additional cri-
terion of impairment. Thus, if a cluster of symptoms leads to significant
suffering or to reduced social functioning then a disorder is diagnosed. The
problem is that epidemiological studies suggest that adolescent depression
is a continuum that is associated with problems at most levels of severity.

Even minor forms of depression are associated with social impairment (Pickles *et al.*, 2001). Indeed, it seems that there is no 'good' level of depression; it is better for an adolescent to have no symptoms of depression at all than to be averagely depressed (Harrington and Clark, 1998). Thus, in the Oregon Adolescent Depression Project the level of psychosocial impairment increased as a direct function of the number of depressive symptoms (Lewinsohn *et al.*, 1998). Moreover, in line with studies of adults (Angst *et al.*, 1997), much of the morbidity associated with depression occurred in the 'milder' but more numerous cases of minor depression. Mild forms of adolescent depression are a risk factor for depression in early adulthood (Pine *et al.*, 1999). The implication is that at least from an epidemiological perspective it is very difficult to draw the line between 'normal' depression and 'depressive disorder'.

The second conceptual issue is that major depression in adolescents usually occurs in conjunction with other psychiatric disorders, particularly conduct disorders and anxiety (Angold *et al.*, 1999*a*). The question therefore arises as to whether depression can be meaningfully differentiated from these other problems in terms of aetiology, course, and response to treatment.

In the present chapter the general perspective will be that depressive disorder is a useful concept in adolescent psychiatry. It tells us things about correlates, treatment, and outcome that broader concepts (such as of 'internalizing disorder') do not. Nevertheless, it is acknowledged from the outset that much more work remains to be done on the validity of the concept of depressive disorder in this age group.

Diagnosis and classification

Most clinicians and researchers use one of the major schemes for diagnosis, DSM-IV or ICD-10 (World Health Organization, 1992; American Psychiatric Association, 1994). The schemes differ in many ways, but at the core of both is the concept of an episodic disorder of varying degrees of severity that is characterized by depressed mood or loss of enjoyment that persists for several weeks. The individual must also experience other symptoms during the episode. These include *depressive thinking* such as pessimism about the future or suicidal ideas, and *biological symptoms* such as early waking, reduced appetite and weight loss.

Subcategorizing adolescent depressive disorder by severity is widely accepted. Both DSM-IV and ICD-10 distinguish between mild, moderate, and severe episodes of depression. The schemes differ, however, in their definitions of severity. In ICD-10 severity is defined by symptoms, whereas in DSM-IV severity is defined in terms of symptoms and functional impairment. In clinical practice impairment is a useful guide both to choice of treatment and to prognosis. For example, adolescents with severe depression, defined as complete disability in one or more domains of social functioning (e.g. unable to go to school), are much less likely to respond to psychological treatment than those with mild or moderate depression (Jayson et al., 1998). Nevertheless, it can be difficult to link impairment to specific symptoms, and there are many cases whose impairment seems out of proportion to their symptoms (Angold et al., 1999c).

Both ICD-10 and DSM-IV distinguish between psychotic and non-psychotic episodes of depression. Psychotic depression is very uncommon before mid-adolescence, but the concept is useful in adults to the extent that it predicts a worse prognosis (Lee and Murray, 1998). Psychotic symptoms also presage worse outcomes in adolescent depression (Strober et al., 1993). The distinction between depression that occurs as part of bipolar disorder and unipolar depression is also useful (Strober, 1992).

Epidemiology

Prevalence

Recent studies have found that the one-year (or less) prevalence of major depressive disorder associated with impairment ranges from around 1 per cent (Simonoff et al., 1997), through 3 per cent (Cohen et al., 1993; Lewinsohn et al., 1998) to 6 per cent (Olsson and von Knorring, 1999). When all kinds of depressive disorders are included, then the prevalence can be as high as 10 per cent (Angold et al., 1998). The cumulative probability of having a depressive disorder by late adolescence seems to be between 10 and 20 per cent (Lewinsohn et al., 1998; Oldehinkel et al., 1999; Olsson and von Knorring, 1999).

Developmental trends and gender differences

Depressive disorder is less common among preadolescent children than among adolescents (Simonoff et al., 1997; Angold et al., 1998; Lewinsohn et al., 1998; Oldehinkel et al., 1999; Olsson and von Knorring, 1999; Meltzer et al., 2000). For instance in a large British national survey the odds of having a depressive disorder for 11- to 15-years-olds compared to 5- to 10-year-olds were 8.5 (Meltzer et al., 2000). The origins of these reliable developmental differences are not well understood, but there are several pointers about possible causes. Age trends in depression are stronger in girls than in boys. Most studies have found that in prepubertal children there is either no gender difference in the prevalence of depression or there is a small male preponderance. In contrast, by late adolescence the female preponderance found in adult depression is well established. The finding that the gender difference seems to be linked more to puberty than to age (Angold *et al.*, 1998) raises important questions about the mechanisms involved. It is possible that there is some direct vulnerability arising from changes in hormone levels, such as androgens (Angold *et al.*, 1999*b*). However, puberty is accompanied by many other changes, such as in cognition and in stressful events. Morever, even in large samples it can be very difficult to tease apart the effects of age and puberty. Probably there are several reasons for the greater vulnerability of girls. Before adolescence, girls are more likely than boys to have risk factors for depression such as certain personality features (Nolen-Hoeksema and Girgus, 1994). However, these risk factors are not sufficient to cause depression until the person experiences the biological and social challenges of adolescence (Nolen-Hoeksema and Girgus, 1994; Cyranowski *et al.*, 2000).

Comorbidity

In a review of around twenty epidemiological studies based on DSM, Angold and colleagues (Angold *et al.*, 1999*a*) found that the most common comorbid disorders were conduct disorder (40 per cent) and anxiety disorders including obsessive-compulsive disorder (34 per cent). This is far greater than would be expected on the basis of the rates of these disorders in the general population.

Longitudinal and epidemiological studies suggest that anxiety tends to precede depression in both adolescents and children (Kovacs *et al.*, 1989) and adults (Merikangas *et al.*, 1996), raising the possibility that depression is in some sense secondary to anxiety. It may be that they share a common temperamental basis, such as emotionality. Genetic studies suggest the possibility of a common genetic diathesis although this may be stronger in the post-pubertal adolescent compared with the pre-pubertal child (Eley and Stevenson, 1999; Rice, Harold *et al.*, 2002).

There are several explanations for comorbidity of depression and conduct disorder. It could be that depression is simply an integral part of conduct disorder. Zoccolillo (Zoccolillo, 1992), for instance, suggested that conduct disorder is a problem of multiple dysfunction, with depression a dysfunction of affect regulation and conduct disorder a dysfunction of social regulation. Alternatively, it may be that conduct disorder causes depression. Adolescents with conduct disorder sometimes behave in ways that increase their risk of the kinds of adverse events that cause depression, such as inconsistent parenting (O'Connor *et al.*, 1998*a*). Another possibility is that they share risk factors. Fergusson *et al.* (1996) reported that much of the correlation between the two could be explained by shared risk factors such as family dysfunction. Some of these shared risk factors may be genetic. O'Connor and coworkers (O'Connor *et al.*, 1998*b*), found that nearly 50 per cent of the association between depression and conduct disorder could be explained by a common genetic liability.

Course and outcome

By comparison with non-depressed subjects, adolescents diagnosed as depressed are more likely to have subsequent episodes of depression. Thus, studies of adolescents meeting DSM-III criteria for depression have shown that depression often recurs. For example, Kovacs *et al.* (1984*a*) found that about 70 per cent of young patients with a major depressive disorder had another episode within five years. This increased risk of recurrence extends into adulthood. Harrington and colleagues (Harrington *et al.*, 1990) followed up sixty-three depressed children and adolescents on average 18 years after their initial contact. The depressed group was four times more likely to have an episode of depression after the age of 17 years than a control group who had been matched on a large number of variables, including non-depressive symptoms. This increased risk was maintained well into adulthood and was associated with significantly increased rates of attending psychiatric services and of using medication, as compared to the controls. A preliminary report from a large follow-up study in the United States has found increased rates of completed suicide in depressed adolescent patients (Rao *et al.*, 1993).

A variety of different factors appear to predict continuity. The characteristics of the index episode are important to the extent that youngsters with 'double depression' (major depression and dysthymic disorder) have a worse short term outcome than those with major depression alone (Kovacs *et al.*, 1984*a*). Older adolescents have a worse prognosis than younger ones, and continuity to adulthood is best predicted by a severe adult-like depressive presentation (Harrington *et al.*, 1990). Although it is often assumed that continuity of depression is mainly due to the direct persistence of the initial disorder or of premorbid psychological and/or biological vulnerabilities to depression, it should be borne in mind that environmental mechanisms may also be involved. For instance, some studies have found that persistence of adverse family environments is an important determinant of relapse (Asarnow *et al.*, 1998). Relapse may also be linked to parental depression. Hammen and co-workers (Hammen *et al.*, 1991) found a close temporal relationship between maternal depression and a recurrence of depression in the young person, supporting the idea of an environmentally mediated mechanism.

Recovery from the index episode

Although the risk of recurrence of juvenile depression is high, it is important to know that the prognosis for the index episode is quite good. The available data suggest that the majority of young people with major depression will recover within two years. For example, Kovacs *et al.* (1984*b*) reported that the cumulative probability of recovery from major depression by one year after onset was 74 per cent and by two years was 92 per cent. This study was based on subjects who in most cases had a previous history of treatment for emotional-behavioural disorder. However, Keller *et al.* (1988) reported very similar findings in a retrospective study of time to recovery from first episode of major depression in young people who had mostly not received treatment. The probability of recovery for adolescent inpatients with major depression also appears to be about 90 per cent by two years (Strober *et al.*, 1993), though those with long-standing depressions recover less quickly than those whose presentation is acute.

It seems, then, that most young people with major depression will recover to a significant extent, but that a minority will have further episodes.

Aetiology

The aetiology of adolescent depressive disorders is likely to be multifactorial, including both genetic and environmental risk factors, which act through psychological and biological processes.

Risk factors

Genetic factors

There is evidence that affective disorders in adults have a genetic component. Genetic influences seem to be the strongest for bipolar disorders (McGuffin and Katz, 1986), but unipolar major depressions also show significant heritability (Kendler *et al.*, 1995). There have thus far been no large systematic twin or adoption studies of depressive disorder in young people. However, family studies find increased rates of depression among relatives of young probands with depressive disorder (Harrington *et al.*, 1993). Moreover twin studies suggest modest genetic influences on depressive symptoms in adolescence (Thapar and McGuffin, 1994; Eaves *et al.*, 1997), though this has not been replicated in adoption studies (Eley *et al.*, 1998). Twin studies also report that some of the stability in depressive symptoms arises from genetic factors (O'Connor *et al.*, 1998c). The mode of inheritance is uncertain, but genetic effects are likely to act through multiple mechanisms, many of which are indirect (Silberg *et al.*, 1999). For example, in some cases it seems that genetic factors act by increasing vulnerability to adverse life events, an example of gene-environment interaction. In others genes appear to increase the liability to depressing life events, such as falling out with friends, an example of active gene-environment correlation (Silberg *et al.*, 1999).

Adversity

It will be appreciated that just because a disorder runs in families, it does not necessarily follow that the linkages are mediated genetically. It is likely that family environmental factors are also important. For instance, discordant intrafamilial relationships seem to be strong predictors of the course of depressive disorders among the young. Young people with depression who have been admitted to hospital who return to families who show high levels of criticism and discord have a much worse outcome than children returning to more harmonious environments (Asarnow *et al.*, 1988).

Stresses and acute life events outside of the family, such as friendship difficulties and bullying, are also likely to be relevant in this age group (Goodyer *et al.*, 1989). Depressive disorders in young people often follow stressful life events (Goodyer *et al.*, 1993) such as parental discord, bullying, and physical, sexual or emotional abuse (Boney-McCoy and Finkelhor, 1996; Kaplan *et al.*, 1998). There is, however, great variation in young people's responses to acute adversity. Most young people who experience such events do not develop depressive disorder (Goodyer, 1990; Silberg *et al.*, 2001). For example, in a longitudinal epidemiological study in New York, 75 per cent of abused or neglected children were free of depression (Brown *et al.*, 1999). Conversely, a significant minority of depressed young people show no obvious acute precipitant for their episode (Goodyer *et al.*, 1993).

Processes

Biological

There has been much research on the biological basis for depression in young people. Over the years this research has produced a range of positive findings, usually of modest size, as well as many negatives. Whilst it is true to say that none of these biological findings distinguishes between depressed and non-depressed people better than clinical assessment, they continue to stimulate ideas about the neurobiology of depression. One of the most promising lines of research has been on stress hormones such as cortisol. It has been known for a long time that the kinds of stresses that are often associated with depression activate the hypothalamic-anterior pituitary-adrenocortical axis. In a prospective study of clinically referred adolescents with major depression Goodyer and colleagues (Goodyer *et al.*, 2001) found that persistence of major depression was linked to continuing adverse events, which were more common in those with persisting cortisol hypersecretion. The implication is that cortisol could mediate the links between adversity and depression.

Another promising line of biological research, which has produced many positive findings, has been on sleep. Sleep is often disturbed in adolescent depression. Like other biological manifestations, the question arises as to how far these changes are simply a consequence of depression and how far a cause. However, the finding from two studies that sleep disturbance may be a predictor of relapse (Goetz *et al.*, 2001; Emslie *et al.*, 2001*a*) suggests that the sleep wake cycle could be directly involved in mood regulation and disorder in adolescents.

One of the challenges for future research will be to link these findings to what is known about the pharmacology of antidepressants. There are however some plausible mechanisms. For example, antidepressants could act upon the neural pathways that control sleep and the hypothalamic-anterior pituitary-adrenocortical axis.

Distorted thinking

In cognitive theory depression is triggered by the perception and cognitive processing of adverse events. Much previous research has shown that depression in young people is associated with negative thinking and some recent studies have reported that such thinking can presage subsequent depression (Cole *et al.*, 2001; Kistner *et al.*, 2001). It will be appreciated however that just because negative cognitions precede depression it does not necessarily follow that they cause it. The mediating effects of cognitions were examined in a randomised trial of cognitive therapy for depression (Kolko *et al.*, 2001). This trial found that although the therapy was effective, its beneficial effects did not depend on changes in cognitions. Thus, although cognitive theory has been an important stimulus for the development of effective therapies, cognitive therapy may work through other processes.

Assessment

Defining the boundaries between extremes of normal behaviour is a dilemma that pervades all of psychiatry. It is especially problematic to establish the limits of depressive disorder in adolescence because of the cognitive and physical changes that take place during this time. Adolescents tend to feel things particularly deeply and mood swings are common during the teenage years. It can be difficult to distinguish these intense emotional reactions from depressive disorder. By contrast, young adolescents do not find it easy to describe how they are feeling and can confuse emotions such as anger and sadness.

Assessment of young people who present with symptoms of depression must therefore begin with the basic question of diagnosis. This will mean interviewing the adolescent alone. It is not enough to rely on accounts obtained from the parents since they may not notice depression in their offspring, and may not even be aware of suicidal attempts. Indeed, it is now common practise to obtain information from several sources. Adolescents usually give a better account of symptoms related to internal experience whereas parents are likely to be better informants on overt behavioural difficulties. Accounts from children and parents are usually supplemented by information from other sources, particularly teachers and direct observations.

Treatment

General principles

Many of the general principles of treatment follow from the description of the depressed young person's difficulties outlined above. Comorbidity is frequent, there are many complications and there is a high risk of relapse. Other types of adversity are part of the cause and may need intervention in their own right. The course is determined by more than just the presence and severity of depression. Therefore, attention must be paid to biological, familial, educational, and peer contributions. As with other child psychiatric disorders, it is important not only to treat the presenting problems but also to foster normal development. A treatment programme therefore has multiple aims: to reduce depression, to treat comorbid disorders, to promote social and emotional adjustment, to improve self-esteem, to relieve family distress, and to prevent relapse.

Pharmacotherapy

Most of the early research on pharmacotherapy was with the tricyclic antidepressants (TCAs). The results from open trials were encouraging but almost all of the randomized controlled double-blind trials found no significant differences between oral tricyclics and placebo (Hazell *et al.*, 1995).

Tricyclics are an effective treatment for adult depression (Boyce and Judd, 1999), raising the question as to the possible explanations of the failure of clinical trials among the young. The first possibility is that the failure is more apparent than real, and stems from some of the methodological issues involved in conducting trials in this age group. For example, consent must in practise be obtained from two people, and many parents are reluctant to allow their children into a study in which one of the treatments is medication. This may be especially difficult in studies involving tricyclics, where regular monitoring of cardiac function is required. The result may have been that particularly severe, and perhaps less responsive, cases of depression have been admitted to the tricyclic trials. There have also been technical problems with some of the trials (Hazell et al., 1995) of which perhaps the most striking is their relatively small sample sizes. Significant drug effects within subgroups could easily have been missed. In addition, some trials have had very high response rates in the group given placebo (Puig-Antich et al., 1987) making it even more difficult to detect an effect of active drug.

The apparent failure of the tricyclic trials has led to great interest in the results of trials with other antidepressants, particularly the serotonin-specific reuptake inhibitors (SSRIs) such as fluoxetine and paroxetine. An early small trial was negative (Simeon et al., 1990) but several subsequent larger trials have produced positive results. The first of these was conducted by Emslie and colleagues (Emslie et al., 1997). The second was a multicentre industry funded study (Keller et al., 2001), in which nearly 300 adolescents aged between 13 and 18 years were randomized to paroxetine (20–40 mg), imipramine, or placebo. The response rates on the Clinical Global Improvement Scale were 66, 52 and 48 per cent respectively, a significant difference in favour of paroxetine. In another industry-sponsored randomized study (Emslie et al., 2001c) more than 200 children and adolescents were randomized to fluoxetine 20 mg daily or placebo. Significantly more fluoxetine (52 per cent) than placebo-treated (37 per cent) patients had a Clinical Global Improvement score of 1 or 2 ($p = 0.028$). Open-label trials with sertraline (Nixon et al., 2001) and citalopram (Bostic et al., 2001) have produced encouraging results.

In cases who remit, how long should antidepressants be continued? In a small ($n = 40$) randomized industry-sponsored trial Emslie and colleagues (Emslie et al., 2001b) reported that the time to relapse was significantly longer in those who continued fluoxetine after recovery from major depression than those who had placebo. These findings require replication in a larger study. In the meantime they suggest it may be sensible to continue SSRIs for at least six months after recovery from depressive disorder.

If there has been no response to the 'standard' dose of an SSRI after a few weeks there may be a case for increasing the dose to the maximum tolerated (Hoog *et al.*, 2001). In patients who fail to respond to an increased dose of SSRI there should be a review of the possible reasons. Non-compliance can be a major issue in this age group, and blood levels (if available) or pill counts may help to identify this problem. There should also be a review of the diagnosis, and of any possible comorbid problems. Undiagnosed abuse, family discord, bipolar disorder, drug dependence or physical illnesses may be important (Brent, 2001).

There are no empirical data to guide the next step. In patients who fail to respond to one SSRI the Texas Consensus Conference recommended a trial of another (Hughes *et al.*, 1999), on the grounds that some of the SSRIs are chemically distinct. If the young person fails to respond to a second SSRI, then monotherapy with another antidepressant should be considered, such as venlafaxine or a tricyclic. Brent (2001) reported that in an open trial around 50 per cent of those who failed to respond to an adequate trial with an SSRI responded to venlafaxine. Failure to respond to a third antidepressant should trigger another review of the clinical state. In many services it would be at this point that other forms of therapy might be considered, such as admission to an inpatient unit. Augmentation with another agent such as lithium or bupropion might also be an option, but only if the patient has derived at least some benefit from the first treatment. Combination treatments can however be associated with toxicity.

An advantage of antidepressants is that because they can be prescribed by psychiatrists, paediatricians and general practitioners, they should be accessible to many young people. This issue is important because epidemiological studies continue to show that many depressed adolescents never receive professional help (Flament *et al.*, 2001; Wu *et al.*, 2001).

The main disadvantages of antidepressants are their side effects. SSRIs seem to have fewer side effects than the tricyclics and, unlike the tricyclics, do not usually require specific cardiovascular monitoring (Gutgesell *et al.*, 1999). However, symptoms such as gastrointestinal upset and sleep disturbance can be a problem and behavioural activation, which includes motor restlessness, is another side effect. Abrupt discontinuation of SSRIs can lead to symptoms such as dizziness, nausea, and lethargy, which may raise parental concerns about 'addiction'. An industry-sponsored discontinuation study with depressed children and adolescents who had been on SSRI for nineteen weeks suggested however that such symptoms did not occur with fluoxetine, which has a long half life (Heiligenstein *et al.*, 2001).

Cognitive-behaviour therapy

Cognitive-behavioural treatment (CBT) programmes were developed to address the cognitive distortions and deficits identified in depressed adolescents (see above). Many varieties of CBT exist for adolescent depression, but they all have the following common characteristics. First, the adolescent is the focus of treatment (although most CBT programmes involve parents). Second, the adolescent and therapist collaborate to solve problems. Third, the therapist teaches the adolescent to monitor and keep a record of thoughts and behaviour. There is therefore emphasis on diary keeping and on homework assignments. Fourth, treatment usually combines several different procedures, including behavioural techniques (such as activity scheduling) and cognitive strategies (such as cognitive restructuring).

A metaanalysis (Harrington *et al.*, 1998*a*) of six randomized trials with clinically diagnosed cases of depressive disorder found that CBT was significantly superior to comparison conditions such as remaining on a waiting list or having relaxation training. However, this metaanalysis noted that CBT had not been used with severe cases of depression nor in cases with many comorbid problems such as conduct disorder or repeated self-harm.

Against this background, the finding that CBT is an effective short term treatment for depressed adolescents with conduct disorder is important. Rohde *et al.* (2001) reported that adolescents with comorbid depression and conduct disorder had lower levels of depression if given the Coping With Depression Course then if they had academic tutoring. Wood and colleagues obtained similarly encouraging results within an equally challenging sample (Wood *et al.*, 2001). They conducted the first randomized trial of treatment for adolescents who repeatedly harm themselves, of whom around 80 per cent had major depression. They found that a group-delivered treatment with many cognitive-behavioural elements led to a lower risk of repetition of self-harm than routine care.

If an adolescent fails to respond to CBT then the reasons for this should be reviewed. It may be that other problems besides depression are present. Review may also indicate some specific reasons for the failure of CBT. For example, CBT is less effective when given by a therapist who tells the patient what to do (Scott, 1998). If CBT has been given to a reasonable standard for eight weeks and there has been no response or the young person is getting worse then a trial of SSRI should be considered.

There are few data regarding the factors that influence treatment outcome. The most consistent finding thus far has been that adolescents with severe depressive disorders respond less well to CBT than those with mild or moderately severe conditions (Clarke *et al.*, 1992; Jayson *et al.*, 1998). For example, Jayson and colleagues found that only a quarter of young people who were unable to function in at least one social domain (e.g. unable to go to school) responded to CBT. Research has also examined the role that changes in negative cognitions might have in predicting outcome. CBT is not differentially more effective in cases with high cognitive distortion (Clarke *et al.*, 1992). Lewinsohn and coworkers (Lewinsohn *et al.*, 1990) found that changes in depressogenic cognitions did not account for the superiority of CBT over remaining on a waiting list.

Although training in cognitive therapy with adults is available in many centres, it can be difficult to get training in cognitive therapy with young people. There is some evidence however that a related individual psychotherapy, interpersonal psychotherapy, can be used successfully by novice therapists who are well supervised (Santor and Kusumakar, 2001). It may not be necessary therefore for therapists to have very long programmes of training.

Family therapy

There are widely differing definitions of the activity of family therapy, but most therapies have the following features in common (Gorell Barnes, 1994). First, they typically involve face to face work with more than one family member. Second, therapeutic work focuses on altering the interactions among family members. Third, practitioners think of improvement at two levels—that of the presenting problem and that of the relationship patterns associated with the problem.

Two kinds of works have been undertaken with the families of depressed adolescents. The first (Lewinsohn *et al.*, 1990; Clarke *et al.*, 1999) consists of parental attendance at a course run in parallel with the adolescent's treatment (Lewinsohn *et al.*, 1996). The aim of the parents' course is to help them promote the adolescent's learning of new skills. Parents also learn problem solving and communication skills. Adolescents and parents practise these skills in joint sessions.

The second approach involves conjoint family work. In this approach the primary focus is usually within the treatment sessions, which aim directly to change family communication patterns and methods of solving problems. The therapist may also help the family to see depression from the relational function it may have within the family.

There have been at least four randomized controlled trials of family therapy in adolescents depression. Two included cases with major depression (Brent *et al.*, 1997; Harrington *et al.*, 1998*b*) and involved a family intervention only. Two examined the value of parental sessions given in parallel with CBT to children diagnosed with either major depression or dysthymic disorder (Lewinsohn *et al.*, 1990; Clarke *et al.*, 1999). The results have thus far been negative.

On present evidence it would be premature however to conclude that family therapy is ineffective in adolescent depression. With just four trials completed thus far, it could be that significant benefits will emerge in future studies. The association between adolescent depression and family dysfunction is so strong that further studies of family interventions are certainly indicated. However, until there is a firmer empirical basis for family therapy, other interventions will be the treatment of choice.

Promoting remission and preventing relapse

Young people with depressive disorders are likely to have another episode and so it is important to consider the need for prophylactic treatments. Research with depressed adults distinguishes between continuation and maintenance treatments.

The idea behind continuation treatments is that although treatment may suppress the acute symptoms of depression, this treatment should continue until the hypothesized underlying episode has finished. There have been no randomized trials of continuation treatments for juvenile depressive disorders. However, data from a non-randomized trial with depressed adolescents suggest that continuing psychological treatment for six months after remission is feasible and may be effective in preventing relapse (Kroll et al., 1996). The treatment given during the acute episode of adolescent depression should therefore be continued until the patient has been free of depression for around six months.

Maintenance treatments have a different objective, which is to prevent the development of a new episode of depression. Research with adult patients suggests that both pharmacotherapy and psychotherapy may reduce the risk of relapse if maintained for several years after the index depressive episode (Frank et al., 1992; Kupfer, 1992). Clearly, such treatments will be very time consuming and expensive. They cannot therefore be contemplated for more than a small minority of depressed young people. Clinical experience suggests that indications for maintenance treatment include a history of highly recurrent depressive disorder, severely handicapping episodes of depression and chronic major depression.

Prevention of depression

There is a strong case, at least in theory, for preventing depression in young people. Once established, depressive disorder can be difficult to treat (see above) and has a high risk of recurrence that extends into adulthood (Fombonne et al., 2001a). Depression is also associated with personality dysfunction later in life (Kasen et al., 2001). Young people with depression and conduct disorder are at particularly high risk of problems in adulthood (Fombonne *et al.*, 2001*b*), when they have high rates of service use and costs (Knapp *et al.*, 2002).

But how can juvenile depression best be prevented? Recent epidemiological studies have produced several findings that may be useful in developing a preventive strategy. The first is that depression seems to be a continuum that is associated with social impairment at most levels of severity, even below the threshold for disorder (see above). The implication is that preventive programmes should include a *universal* element that targets all people, because a small reduction in morbidity for many individuals could lead to a large reduction in impairment for the population as a whole. The second finding is that juvenile depression has several robust risk factors. These include a family history of depression (Klein *et al.*, 2001), depressive symptoms, a history of other psychiatric disorders such as anxiety (Woodward and Fergusson, 2001), and adverse events such as bereavement (Harrison and Harrington, 2001). Prevention programmes should therefore also include *selective* components that target these high risk groups. Incidentally, although genetic studies suggest that liability to depression is partly inherited, genetic influences often act through increasing susceptibility to adversity (Silberg *et al.*, 2001). The effects of genes are probably not deterministic and so strategies that target environmental mechanisms are not necessarily incompatible with a disorder that has significant heritability.

It follows that a comprehensive preventive strategy should include both universal programmes that include everyone and targeted interventions for high risk groups.

Efficacy of universal programmes

Typically, universal programmes involve either attempts to reduce levels of depression directly or efforts to develop strengths that might protect against depression. Early results with universal depression reduction programmes were not encouraging (Clarke *et al.*, 1993) but recent findings have been a little more promising (Lowry-Webster *et al.*, 2001; Merry *et al.*, 2001). Merry *et al.* (2001), for instance, reported that adolescents given a cognitive-behavioural therapy (CBT) programme delivered through schools had lower levels of depression than adolescents who did not have such a programme.

Depression-focused universal approaches can potentially produce large reductions in depressive symptoms, but their focus on psychopathology can make them unattractive to young people. Another approach is to use interventions that develop positive skills that will not only protect the youngster against depression but may also help them in other domains of development.

An example is the Problem Solving for Life (PSFL) programme, which was evaluated by Spence and colleagues (Spence and Sheffield, 2001). This programme is administered by teachers on a whole classroom basis and involves the learning of problem solving skills. Early results from a controlled study showed reductions in depressive symptoms for high risk students, though these improvements were not maintained at follow-up. A similar approach, which involves students building up strengths, has also produced encouraging preliminary results (Shochet et al., 2001).

Efficacy of targeted programmes

Targeted programmes can be divided into symptom-centred, family history-centred, and event-centred.

Symptom-centred programmes target young people with high scores on depression questionnaires. There is much evidence that cognitive-behavioural programmes run in schools can be effective in reducing depressive symptoms (Harrington et al., 1998c). However, these programmes can be difficult to sustain within educational systems that have many other priorities. There has therefore been interest in applying CBT programmes in non-educational settings. Hamilton et al. (2001) studied the effects of a programme in a primary care setting, a health maintenance organization. Preliminary results from a randomized trial suggested that while the programme had little benefit in 11- and 12-year-olds with low levels of depression, it did seem to help in those with high levels of initial symptoms.

A variety of different approaches are available for the prevention of depression in the offspring of depressed parents (Beardslee and Gladstone, 2001). One of the most promising is the programme used by Clarke and colleagues (Clarke et al., 2001) in a study of the adolescent offspring of depressed parents ascertained through health maintenance organizations. Adolescents were selected because of subdiagnostic depressive symptoms and randomly allocated to routine care or routine care plus a fifteen-session CBT programme. The cumulative incidence of major depression in the CBT group (9 per cent) was significantly less than in the usual care condition (29 per cent).

Many kinds of adverse events increase the risk of depression in young people. Some of these events may be preventable. For instance, a recent review suggested that prevention of child abuse and neglect through parenting programmes of one kind or another could reduce the prevalence of antisocial behaviour in youth (MacMillan, 2001). The same may be true for depression. For other kinds of events, preventive programmes can help young people and their families to deal with the consequences of this event. Sandler and colleagues (Sandler et al., 2001), for example, developed a theoretically based preventive intervention for parentally bereaved youngsters. A randomized trial found that the intervention improved parenting, coping and parental mental health not only immediately afterwards but also at follow-up eleven months later.

Whilst the results from this new wave of prevention trials are encouraging a number of challenges remain. First, the take-up for many depression prevention programmes is relatively poor, and in many cases less than 50 per cent (Harrington *et al.*, 1998*c*). Second, preventive programmes have not thus far been widely translated into routine practise. It is still relatively uncommon, for example, to find that preventive programmes are well established in schools. This is likely to be for a number of reasons, not the least of which are the difficulties in justifying the funds for prevention when in many areas there are scarcely enough resources to treat young people with established mental disorders. Of course, it is often argued that prevention programmes will ultimately save money because fewer people with established disorders will need expensive clinical services. However, the study of Hamilton and colleagues (Hamilton *et al.*, 2001) found that young people in the depression prevention programme tended to make more mental health visits than those who were not. The implication is that prevention programmes are not necessarily cost-effective. Their main justification is humanitarian, not economic.

Conclusions

There is now consistent evidence that depressive disorders in young people are associated with significant impairment, such as poor peer relationships and impaired academic performance. Moreover, there is a significant risk of relapse, which may extend into adult life. Severe depression is not, then, 'normal' or something that adolescents will naturally grow out of. It can be a serious disorder that requires psychiatric treatment.

Research on aetiology suggests that both genetic and environmental factors are important in causing depression among the young. This research has implications for preventive programmes. For example, much of the psychopathological risk to the children of depressed mothers seems to stem from factors other than maternal depression (Goodman and Gotlib, 1999), such as chronic parenting problems. See Chapter 1 for a detailed discussion of parent–child relations and depressive risk in the pre-school child. Future preventive studies probably need to target these factors at least as much as they do parental depression.

For the foreseeable future, however, it will not be possible to prevent more than a small number of cases of juvenile depression. Many challenges remain in the development of effective treatments for established depressive disorders, of which four stand out. First, although several promising treatments have been developed for the acute episode, we know very little about their relative demerits and merits. For example, a key question for future research is how individual psychological treatments compare with the SSRIs. Second, there needs to be greater appreciation of the limitations of current designs for clinical practice. Much extant research has been based on selected samples of cases with only moderately severe depression and without the comorbid problems that often complicate the cases that are seen in everyday practice. 'Pragmatic' studies (Hotopf *et al.*, 1999) with large samples of the kinds of patients who present in routine clinical practice are also required. In particular, information is needed on the efficacy of treatments within severely impaired samples. Third, there needs to be a continuation of efforts to develop and test the kinds of clinical algorithms that are used in routine practice. Treatment researchers have, up to now, tended to conceptualise an intervention as just one treatment modality given for a short time. This strategy has been a necessary first step in the development of coherent, theory driven interventions. The complexity of factors that precipitate and maintain juvenile depression suggests, however, that it is unlikely that any single treatment will be effective in all cases. 'Treatment' in research studies needs therefore to be conceptualised more often as a programme of interventions used singly or in combination that will often follow one after the other, depending on the likely causes of the young person's problems and response to treatment. Finally, there has been little attention so far to ways of preventing relapse or other complications such as suicidal behaviour. Perhaps the most daunting challenge for the future will be to develop better ways of identifying and helping the significant minority of depressed young people in whom their first episode of depression presages further serious psychopathology.

Acknowledgements

Thanks are due to the National Coordinating Centre for Health Technology Assessment, who currently support two randomised trials of treatment for severe mental disorders in adolescence in which RH is involved. The views and opinions expressed herein do not necessarily reflect those of this body.

References

American Psychiatric Association (1987). *Diagnostic and Statistical Manual of Mental Disorders—DSM-III-R. (3rd edition—revised).* American Psychiatric Association, Washington, DC.

American Psychiatric Association (1994). *Diagnostic and Statistical Manual of Mental Disorders—DSM-IV. (4th edition).* American Psychiatric Association, Washington, DC.

Angold, A., Costello, E.J., and Erkanli, A. (1999*a*). Comorbidity. *Journal of Child Psychology and Psychiatry*, **40**, 57–87.

Angold, A., Costello, E.J., Erkanli, A., and Worthman, C.M. (1999*b*). Pubertal changes in hormone levels and depression in girls. *Psychological Medicine*, **29**, 1043–1053.

Angold, A., Costello, E.J., Farmer, E.M.Z., Burns, B.J., and Erkanli, A. (1999*c*). Impaired but undiagnosed. *Journal of the American Academy of Child and Adolescent Psychiatry*, **38**, 129–137.

Angold, A., Costello, E.J., and Worthman, C.M. (1998). Puberty and depression: the roles of age, pubertal status and pubertal timing. *Psychological Medicine*, **28**, 51–61.

Angst, J., Merikangas, K.R., and Preisig, M. (1997). Subthreshold syndromes of depression and anxiety in the community. *Journal of Clinical Psychiatry*, **58** (Suppl. 8), 6–10.

Asarnow, J.R., Goldstein, M.J., Carlson, G.A., Perdue, S., Bates, S., and Keller, J. (1988). Childhood-onset depressive disorders. A follow-up study of rates of rehospitalization and out-of-home placement among child psychiatric inpatients. *Journal of Affective Disorders*, **15**, 245–253.

Beardslee, W. and Gladstone, T.R. (2001). Prevention of childhood depression: recent findings and future prospects. *Biological Psychiatry*, **49**, 1101–1110.

Boney-McCoy, S. and Finkelhor, D. (1996). Is youth victimization related to trauma symptoms and depression after controlling for prior symptoms and family relationships? A longitudinal, prospective study. *Journal of Consulting and Clinical Psychology*, **64**, 1406–1416.

Bostic, J.Q., Prince, J., Brown, K., and Place, S. (2001). A retrospective study of citalopram in adolescents with depression. *Journal of Child and Adolescent Psychopharmacology*, **11**, 131–142.

Boyce, P. and Judd, F. (1999). The place for the tricyclic antidepressants in the treatment of depression. *Australian & New Zealand Journal of Psychiatry*, **33**, 323–327.

Brent, D., Holder, D., Kolko, D., Birmaher, B., Baugher, M., Roth, C., Iyengar, S., and Johnson, B. (1997). A clinical psychotherapy trial for adolescent depression comparing cognitive, family, and supportive treatments. *Archives of General Psychiatry*, **54**, 877–885.

Brent, D.A. (2001). In S. Villani (Ed.), *Scientific Proceedings of the 48th Annual Meeting of the American Academy of Child and Adolescent Psychiatry.* American Academy of Child and Adolescent Psychiatry, Washington, p. 9.

Brown, J., Cohen, P., Johnson, J.G., and Smailes, E.M. (1999). Childhood abuse and neglect: specificity of effects on adolescent and young adult depression and suicidality. *Journal of the American Academy of Child and Adolescent Psychiatry*, **38**, 1490–1496.

Clarke, G., Hornbrook, M., Lynch, F., Polen, M., Gale, J., Beardslee, W., O'Connor, E., and Seeley, J. (2001). In S. Villani (Ed.), *Scientific Proceedings of the 48th Annual Meeting of the American Academy of Child and Adolescent Psychiatry*. American Academy of Child and Adolescent Psychiatry, Washington, p. 94.

Clarke, G.N., Hawkins, W., Murphy, M., and Sheeber, L. (1993). School-based primary prevention of depressive symptomatology in adolescents. Findings from two studies. *Journal of Adolescent Research*, **8**, 183–204.

Clarke, G.N., Hops, H., Lewinsohn, P.M., Andrews, J.A., Seeley, J.R., and Williams, J.A. (1992). Cognitive-behavioral group treatment of adolescent depression: prediction of outcome. *Behavior Therapy*, **23**, 341–354.

Clarke, G.N., Rohde, P., Lewinsohn, P.M., Hops, H., and Seeley, J.R. (1999). Cognitive-behavioural treatment of adolescent depression: efficacy of acute group treatment and booster sessions. *Journal of the American Academy of Child and Adolescent Psychiatry*, **38**, 272–279.

Cohen, P., Cohen, J., Kasen, S., Velez, C.N., Hartmark, C., Johnson, J., Rojas, M., Brook, J., and Streuning, E.L. (1993). An epidemiological study of disorders in late childhood and adolescence—I. Age- and gender-specific prevalence. *Journal of Child Psychology and Psychiatry*, **34**, 851–867.

Cole, D.A., Jacqez, F.M., and Maschman, T.L. (2001). Social origins of depressive cognitions: a longitudinal study of self-perceived competence in children. *Cognitive Therapy and Research*, **25**, 377–395.

Cyranowski, J.M., Frank, E., Young, E., and Shear, K. (2000). Adolescent onset of the gender difference in lifetime rates of major depression. *Archives of General Psychiatry*, **57**, 21–27.

Eaves, L.J., Silberg, J.L., Meyer, J.M., Maes, H.H., Simonoff, E., Pickles, A., Rutter, M., Reynolds, C.A., Heath, A.C., Truett, K.R., Neale, M.C., Erikson, M.T., Loeber, R., and Hewitt, J.K. (1997). Genetics and developmental psychopathology: 2. The main effects of genes and environment on behavioral problems in the Virginia twin study of adolescent behavioral development. *Journal of Child Psychology and Psychiatry*, **38**, 965–980.

Eley, T.C., Deater-Deckard, K., Fombonne, E., Fulker, D.W., and Plomin, R. (1998). An adoption study of depressive symptoms in middle childhood. *Journal of Child Psychology and Psychiatry*, **39**, 337–345.

Eley, T.C. and Stevenson, J. (1999). Exploring the covariation between anxiety and depression symptoms: a genetic analysis of the effects of age and sex. *Journal of Child Psychology and Psychiatry*, **40**, 1273–1282.

Emslie, G., Rush, A., Weinberg, W., Kowatch, R., Hughes, C., Carmody, T., and Rintelmann, J. (1997). A double-blind, randomized placebo-controlled trial of fluoxetine in depressed children and adolescents. *Archives of General Psychiatry*, **54**, 1031–1037.

Emslie, G.J., Armitage, R., Weinberg, W.A., Rush, A.J., Mayes, T.L., and Hoffmann, R.F. (2001*a*). Sleep polysomnography as a predictor of recurrence in children and adolescents with major depression. *International Journal of Neuropsychopharmacology*, 4, 159–168.

Emslie, G.J., Heiligenstein, J.H., Hoog, S.L., Ernest, D., VanHoy, B., Nilsson, M.E., and Jacobson, J.G. (2001b). In S. Villani (Ed.), *Scientific Proceedings of the 48th Annual Meeting of the American Academy of Child and Adolescent Psychiatry*. American Academy of Child and Adolescent Psychiatry, Washington, p. 109.

Emslie, G.J., Heiligenstein, J.H., Wagner, K.D., Bangs, M.E., Hoog, S.L., Brown, E.B., Nilsson, M.E., and Jacobson, J.G. (2001c). In S. Villani (Ed.), *Scientific Proceedings of the 48th Annual Meeting of the American Academy of Child and Adolescent Psychiatry*. American Academy of Child and Adolescent Psychiatry, Washington, p. 108.

Fergusson, D.M., Lynskey, M.T., and Horwood, L.J. (1996). Origins of comorbidity between conduct and affective disorders. *Journal of the American Academy of Child and Adolescent Psychiatry*, 35, 451–460.

Flament, M.F., Cohen, D., Choquet, M., Jeammet, P., and Ledoux, S. (2001). Phenomenology, psychosocial correlates, and treatment seeking in major depression and dysthymia of adolescence. *Journal of the American Academy of Child and Adolescent Psychiatry*, 40, 1070–1078.

Fombonne, E., Wostear, G., Cooper, V., Harrington, R., and Rutter, M. (2001a). The Maudsley long-term follow-up of child and adolescent depression: I. Psychiatric outcomes in adulthood. *British Journal of Psychiatry*, 179, 210–217.

Fombonne, E., Wostear, G., Cooper, V., Harrington, R., and Rutter, M. (2001b). The Maudsley long-term follow-up of child and adolescent depression: II. Suicidality, criminality and social dysfunction in adulthood. *British Journal of Psychiatry*, 179, 218–223.

Frank, E., Kupfer, D.J., Hamer, T., Grochocinski, V.J., and McEachran, A.B. (1992). Maintenance treatment and psychobiologic correlates of endogenous subtypes. *Journal of Affective Disorders*, 25, 181–190.

Goetz, R.R., Wolk, S.I., Coplan, J.D., Ryan, N.D., and Weissman, M.M. (2001). Premorbid polysomnographic signs in depressed adolescents: a reanalysis of EEG sleep after longitudinal follow-up in adulthood. *Biological Psychiatry*, 49, 930–942.

Goodman, S.H. and Gotlib, I.H. (1999). Risk for psychopathology in the children of depressed mothers: a developmental model for understanding mechanisms of transmission. *Psychological Review*, 106, 458–490.

Goodyer, I.M. (1990). *Life Experiences, Development and Childhood Psychopathology*. John Wiley, Chichester.

Goodyer, I.M., Cooper, P.J., Vize, C., and Ashby, L. (1993). Depression in 11 to 16 year old girls: the role of past parental psychopathology and exposure to recent life events. *Journal of Child Psychology and Psychiatry*, 34, 1103–1115.

Goodyer, I.M., Park, R.J., and Herbert, J. (2001). Psychosocial and endocrine features of chronic first-episode major depression in 8–16 year olds. *Biological Psychiatry*, 50, 351–357.

Goodyer, I.M., Wright, C., and Altham, P.M.E. (1989). Recent friendships in anxious and depressed school-age children. *Psychological Medicine*, **19**, 165–174.

Gorell Barnes, G. (1994). In M. Rutter, E. Taylor, and L. Hersov (Eds.), *Child and Adolescent Psychiatry: Modern Approaches. (3rd Edition)* Blackwell Scientific, Oxford, pp. 946–965.

Gutgesell, H., Atkins, D., Barst, R., Buck, M., Franklin, W., Humes, R., Ringel, R., Shaddy, R., and Taubert, K.A. (1999). AHA scientific statement: cardiovascular monitoring of children and adolescents receiving psychotropic drugs. *Journal of the American Academy of Child and Adolescent Psychiatry*, **38**, 1047–1050.

Hamilton, J.D., Gillham, J., Patton, K., and Freres, D. (2001). In S. Villani (Ed.), *Scientific Proceedings of the 48th Annual Meeting of the American Academy of Child and Adolescent Psychiatry*. American Academy of Child and Adolescent Psychiatry, Washington, p. 95.

Hammen, C., Burge, D., and Adrian, C. (1991). Timing of mother and child depression in a longitudinal study of children at risk. *Journal of Consulting and Clinical Psychology*, **59**, 341–345.

Harrington, R., Whittaker, J., Shoebridge, P., and Campbell, F. (1998*a*). Systematic review of efficacy of cognitive behaviour therapies in child and adolescent depressive disorder. *British Medical Journal*, **316**, 1559–1563.

Harrington, R.C. and Clark, A. (1998). Prevention and early intervention for depression in adolescence and early adult life. *European Archives of Psychiatry and Clinical Neuroscience*, **248**, 32–45.

Harrington, R.C., Fudge, H., Rutter, M., Bredenkamp, D., Groothues, C., and Pridham, J. (1993). Child and adult depression: a test of continuities with data from a family study. *British Journal of Psychiatry*, **162**, 627–633.

Harrington, R.C., Fudge, H., Rutter, M., Pickles, A., and Hill, J. (1990). Adult outcomes of childhood and adolescent depression: I. Psychiatric status. *Archives of General Psychiatry*, **47**, 465–473.

Harrington, R.C., Kerfoot, M., Dyer, E., McNiven, F., Gill, J., Harrington, V., Woodham, A., and Byford, S. (1998*b*). Randomized trial of a home based family intervention for children who have deliberately poisoned themselves. *Journal of the American Academy of Child and Adolescent Psychiatry*, **37**, 512–518.

Harrington, R.C., Whittaker, J., and Shoebridge, P. (1998*c*). Psychological treatment of depression in children and adolescents: a review of treatment research. *British Journal of Psychiatry*, **173**, 291–298.

Harrison, L. and Harrington, R. (2001). Adolescents' bereavement experiences. Prevalence, association with depression and use of services. *Journal of Adolescence*, **24**, 159–169.

Hazell, P., O'Connell, D., Heathcote, D., Robertson, J., and Henry, D. (1995). Efficacy of tricyclic drugs in treating child and adolescent depression: a meta-analysis. *British Medical Journal*, **310**, 897–901.

Heiligenstein, J.H., Hoog, S.L., Nilsson, M.E., and Jacobson, J.G. (2001). In S. Villani (Ed.), *Scientific Proceedings of the 48th Annual Meeting of the American*

Academy of Child and Adolescent Psychiatry. American Academy of Child and Adolescent Psychiatry, Washington, p. 115.

Hoog, S.L., Heiligenstein, J.H., Wagner, K.D., Findling, R., Ernest, D., Nilsson, M.E., Brown, E., and Jacobson, J.G. (2001). In S. Villani (Ed.), *Scientific Proceedings of the 48th Annual Meeting of the American Academy of Child and Adolescent Psychiatry.* American Academy of Child and Adolescent Psychiatry, Washington, p. 114.

Hotopf, M., Churchill, R., and Lewis, G. (1999). Pragmatic randomized controlled trials in psychiatry. *British Journal of Psychiatry,* **175,** 217–223.

Hughes, C.W., Emslie, G.J., Crimson, M.L., Wagner, K.D., Birmaher, B., Geller, B., Pliszka, S.R., Ryan, N.D., Strober, M., Trivedi, M.H., Toprac, M.G., Sedillo, A., Llana, M.E., Lopez, M., Rush, A.J., and The Texas Consensus Conference Panel on Medication Treatment of Childhood Major Depressive Disorder (1999). The Texas Children's Medication Algorithm Project: report of the Texas Consensus Conference Panel on Medication Treatment of Childhood Major Depressive Disorder. *Journal of the American Academy of Child and Adolescent Psychiatry,* **38,** 1442–1454.

Jayson, D., Wood, A.J., Kroll, L., Fraser, J., and Harrington, R.C. (1998). Which depressed patients respond to cognitive-behavioral treatment? *Journal of the American Academy of Child and Adolescent Psychiatry,* **37,** 35–39.

Kaplan, S.J., Pelcovitz, D., Salzinger, S., Weiner, M., Mandel, F.S., Lesser, M.L., and Labruna, V.E. (1998). Adolescent physical abuse: risk for adolescent psychiatric disorders. *American Journal of Psychiatry,* **155,** 954–959.

Kasen, S., Cohen, P., Skodol, A.E., Johnson, G., Smailes, E., and Brook, J.S. (2001). Childhood depression and adult personality disorder: alternative pathways of continuity. *Archives of General Psychiatry,* **58,** 231–236.

Keller, M.B., Beardslee, W., Lavori, P.W., Wunder, J., Drs, D.L., and Samuelson, H. (1988). Course of major depression in non-referred adolescents: a retrospective study. *Journal of Affective Disorders,* **15,** 235–243.

Keller, M.B., Ryan, N.D., Strober, M., Klein, R.G., Kutcher, S.P., Birmaher, B., Hagino, O.R., Koplewicz, H., Carlson, G.A., Clarke, G.N., Emslie, G.J., Feinberg, D., Geller, B., Kusumakar, V., Papatheodorou, G., Sack, W.H., Sweeney, M., Wagner, K.D., Weller, E.B., Winters, N.C., Oakes, R., and McCafferty, J.P. (2001). Efficacy of paroxetine in the treatment of adolescent major depression: a randomized, controlled trial. *Journal of the American Academy of Child and Adolescent Psychiatry,* **40,** 762–772.

Kendler, K.S., Kessler, R.C., Walters, E.E., MacLean, C., Neale, M.C., Heath, A.C., and Eaves, L.J. (1995). Stressful life events, genetic liability, and onset of an episode of major depression in women. *American Journal of Psychiatry,* **152,** 833–842.

Kistner, J.A., Ziergert, D.I., Castro, R., and Robertson, B. (2001). Helplessness in early childhood: prediction of symptoms associated with depression and negative self-worth. *Merrill-Palmer Quarterly,* **47,** 336–354.

Klein, D.N., Lewinsohn, P.M., Seeley, J.R., and Rohde, P. (2001). A family study of major depressive disorder in a community sample of adolescents. *Archives of General Psychiatry*, **58**, 13–20.

Knapp, M., McCrone, P., Fombonne, E., Beecham, J., and Wostear, G. (2002). The Maudsley long-term follow-up of child and adolescent depression. *British Journal of Psychiatry*, **180**, 19–23.

Kolko, D.J., Brent, D.A., Baugher, M., Bridge, J., and Birmaher, B. (2001). Cognitive and family therapies for adolescent depression: treatment specificity, mediation, and moderation. *Journal of Consulting and Clinical Psychology*, **68**, 603–614.

Kovacs, M., Feinberg, T.L., Crouse-Novak, M., Paulauskas, S.L., Pollock, M., and Finkelstein, R. (1984a). Depressive disorders in childhood. II. A longitudinal study of the risk for a subsequent major depression. *Archives General Psychiatry*, **41**, 643–649.

Kovacs, M., Feinberg, T.L., Crouse-Novak, M.A., Paulauskas, S.L., and Finkelstein, R. (1984b). Depressive disorders in childhood. I. A longitudinal prospective study of characteristics and recovery. *Archives of General Psychiatry*, **41**, 229–237.

Kovacs, M., Gatsonis, C., Paulauskas, S., and Richards, C. (1989). Depressive disorders in childhood. IV. A longitudinal study of comorbidity with and risk for anxiety disorders. *Archives of General Psychiatry*, **46**, 776–782.

Kroll, L., Harrington, R.C., Gowers, S., Frazer, J., and Jayson, D. (1996). Continuation of cognitive-behavioural treatment in adolescent patients who have remitted from major depression. Feasibility and comparison with historical controls. *Journal of the American Academy of Child and Adolescent Psychiatry*, **35**, 1156–1161.

Kupfer, D. (1992). Maintenance treatment in recurrent depression: current and future directions. *British Journal of Psychiatry*, **161**, 309–316.

Lee, A.S. and Murray, R.M. (1988). The long-term outcome of Maudsley depressives. *British Journal of Psychiatry*, **153**, 741–751.

Lewinsohn, P.M., Clarke, G.N., Hops, H., and Andrews, J. (1990). Cognitive-behavioural treatment for depressed adolescents. *Behavior Therapy*, **21**, 385–401.

Lewinsohn, P.M., Clarke, G.N., Rohde, P., Hops, H., and Seeley, J.R. (1996). In E. Hibbs and P.S. Jensen (Eds.), *Psychosocial Treatments for Child and Adolescent Disorders. Empirically Based Strategies for Clinical Practice*. American Psychological Association, Washington, DC, pp. 109–135.

Lewinsohn, P.M., Rohde, P., and Seeley, J.R. (1998). Major depressive disorder in older adolescents: prevalence, risk factors, and clinical implications. *Clinical Psychology Review*, **18**, 765–794.

Lowry-Webster, H.M., Barrett, P.M., and Dadds, M.R. (2001). A universal prevention trial of anxiety and depressive symptomatology in childhood: preliminary data from an Australian study. *Behaviour Change*, **187**, 36–50.

MacMillan, H. (2001). In S. Villani (Ed.), *Scientific Proceedings of the 48th Annual Meeting of the American Academy of Child and Adolescent Psychiatry*. American Academy of Child and Adolescent Psychiatry, Washington, p. 84.

McGuffin, P. and Katz, R. (1986). In J.F.W. Deakin (Ed.), *The Biology of Depression*. Royal College of Psychiatrists, London, pp. 26–52.

Meltzer, H., Gatward, R., Goodman, R., and Ford, T. (2000). *Mental Health of Children and Adolescents in Great Britain*. The Stationery Office, London.

Merikangas, K.R., Angst, J., Eaton, W., Canino, G., Rubio-Stipec, M., Wacker, H., Wittchen, H.U., Andrade, L., Essau, C., Whitaker, A., Kraemer, H., Robins, L.N., and Kupfer, D.J. (1996). Comorbidity and boundaries of affective disorders with anxiety disorders and substance misuse: results of an international task force. *British Journal of Psychiatry—Supplement*, **30**, 58–67.

Merry, S.N., McDowell, H., Wild, C.J., Muller, N., and Bir, J. (2001). In S. Villani (Ed.), *Scientific Proceedings of the 48th Annual Meeting of the American Academy of Child and Adolescent Psychiatry*. American Academy of Child and Adolescent Psychiatry, Washington, p. 95.

Nixon, M.K., Milin, R., Simeon, J.G., Cloutier, P., and Spenst, W. (2001). Sertraline effects in adolescent major depression and dysthymia: a six-month open trial. *Journal of Child and Adolescent Psychopharmacology*, **11**, 131–142.

Nolen-Hoeksema, S. and Girgus, J.S. (1994). The emergence of gender differences in depression during adolescence. *Psychological Bulletin*, **115**, 424–443.

O'Connor, T.G., Deater-Deckard, K., Fulker, D., Rutter, M., and Plomin, R. (1998*a*). Genotype-environment correlations in late childhood and early adolescence: antisocial behavioral problems and coercive parenting. *Developmental Psychology*, **34**, 970–981.

O'Connor, T.G., McGuire, S., Reiss, D., Hetherington, E.M., and Plomin, R. (1998*b*). Co-occurrence of depressive symptoms and antisocial behavior in adolescence: a common genetic liability. *Journal of Abnormal Psychology*, **107**, 27–37.

O'Connor, T.G., Neiderhiser, J.M., Reiss, D., Hetherington, E.M., and Plomin, R. (1998*c*). Genetic contributions to continuity, change, and co-occurrence of antisocial and depressive symptoms in adolescence. *Journal of Child Psychology and Psychiatry*, **39**, 323–336.

Oldehinkel, A.J., Wittchen, H.U., and Schuster, P. (1999). Prevalence, 20-month incidence and outcome of unipolar depressive disorders in a community sample of adolescents. *Psychological Medicine*, **29**(3), 655–658.

Olsson, G.I. and von Knorring, A.L. (1999). Adolescent depression: prevalence in Swedish high-school students. *Acta Psychiatrica Scandinavica*, **99**, 324–331.

Pearce, J.B. (1978). The recognition of depressive disorder in children. *Journal of the Royal Society of Medicine*, **71**, 494–500.

Pickles, A., Rowe, R., Simonoff, E., Foley, D., Rutter, M., and Silberg, J. (2001). Child psychiatric symptoms and psychosocial impairment: relationship and prognostic significance. *British Journal of Psychiatry*, **179**, 230–235.

Pine, D.S., Cohen, E., Cohen, P., and Brook, J. (1999). Adolescent depressive symptoms as predictors of adult depression: moodiness or mood disorder? *American Journal of Psychiatry*, **156**, 133–135.

Puig-Antich, J. (1982). Major depression and conduct disorder in prepuberty. *Journal of the American Academy of Child and Adolescent Psychiatry*, **21**, 118–128.

Puig-Antich, J., Perel, J.M., Lupatkin, W., Chambers, W.J., Tabrizi, M.A., King, J., Goetz, R., Davies, M., and Stiller, R.L. (1987). Imipramine in prepubertal major depressive disorders. *Archives of General Psychiatry*, **44**, 81–89.

Rao, U., Weissman, M.M., Martin, J.A., and Hammond, R.W. (1993). Childhood depression and risk of suicide: preliminary report of a longitudinal study. *Journal of the American Academy of Child and Adolescent Psychiatry*, **32**, 21–27.

Rohde, P., Clarke, G., Mace, D., Jorgensen, J., and Seeley, J. (2001). In S. Villani (Ed.), *Scientific Proceedings of the 48th Annual Meeting of the American Academy of Child and Adolescent Psychiatry*. American Academy of Child and Adolescent Psychiatry, Washington, p. 109.

Sandler, I., Ayers, T., Wolchik, S., and Tein, J. (2001). In S. Villani (Ed.), *Scientific Proceedings of the 48th Annual Meeting of the American Academy of Child and Adolescent Psychiatry*. American Academy of Child and Adolescent Psychiatry, Washington, p. 92.

Santor, D.A. and Kusumakar, V. (2001). Open trial of interpersonal therapy in adolescents with moderate to severe major depression: effectiveness of novice IPT therapists. *Journal of the American Academy of Child and Adolescent Psychiatry*, **40**, 236–240.

Scott, J.M.S. (1998). Cognitive therapy training for psychiatrists. *Advances in Psychiatric Treatment*, **4**, 3–9.

Shochet, I.M., Dadds, M.R., Holland, D., Whitefield, K., Harnett, P.H., and Osgarby, S.M. (2001). The efficacy of a universal school-based program to prevent adolescent depression. *Journal of Clinical Child Psychology*, **30**, 303–315.

Silberg, J., Pickles, A., Rutter, M., Hewitt, J., Simonoff, E., Maes, H., Carbonneau, R., Murrelle, L., Foley, D., and Eaves, L. (1999). The influence of genetic factors and life stress on depression among adolescent girls. *Archives of General Psychiatry*, **56**, 225–232.

Silberg, J., Rutter, M., Neale, M., and Eaves, L. (2001). Genetic moderation of environmental risk for depression and anxiety in adolescent girls. *British Journal of Psychiatry*, **179**, 116–121.

Simeon, J.G., Dinicola, V.F., Ferguson, H.B., and Copping, W. (1990). Adolescent depression: a placebo-controlled fluoxetine treatment study and follow-up. *Progress in Neuro-Psychopharmacology and Biological Psychiatry*, **14**, 791–795.

Simonoff, E., Pickles, A., Meyer, J.M., Silberg, J.L., Maes, H.H., Loeber, R., Rutter, M., Hewitt, J.K., and Eaves, L.J. (1997). The Virginia twin study of adolescent behavioral development. Influences of age, sex, and impairment on rates of disorder. *Archives of General Psychiatry*, **54**, 801–808.

Spence, H. and Sheffield, J. (2001). In S. Villani (Ed.), *Scientific Proceedings of the 48th Annual Meeting of the American Academy of Child and Adolescent Psychiatry*, American Academy of Child and Adolescent Psychiatry, Washington, p. 95.

Strober, M. (1992). In M. Shafii and S.L. Shafii (Eds.), *Clinical Guide to Depression in Children and Adolescents*, American Psychiatric Press, Washington, DC, pp. 251–268.

Strober, M., Lampert, C., Schmidt, S., and Morrell, W. (1993). The course of major depressive disorder in adolescents: I. Recovery and risk of manic switching in a 24-month prospective, naturalistic follow-up of psychotic and nonpsychotic subtypes. *Journal of the American Academy of Child and Adolescent Psychiatry*, **32**, 34–42.

Thapar, A. and McGuffin, P. (1994). A twin study of depressive symptoms in childhood. *British Journal of Psychiatry*, **165**, 259–265.

Weinberg, W.A., Rutman, J., Sullivan, L., Penick, E.C., and Dietz, S.G. (1973). Depression in children referred to an educational diagnostic centre: diagnosis and treatment. *Journal of Paediatrics*, **83**, 1065–1072.

Wood, A., Trainor, G., Rothwell, J., Moore, A., and Harrington, R.C. (2001). Randomized trial of group therapy for repeated deliberate self-harm in adolescents. *Journal of the American Academy of Child and Adolescent Psychiatry*, **40**, 1246–1253.

Woodward, L.J. and Fergusson, D.M. (2001). Life course outcomes of young people with anxiety disorders in adolescence. *Journal of the American Academy of Child and Adolescent Psychiatry*, **40**, 1086–1093.

World Health Organization (1992). *The ICD-10 Classification of Mental and Behavioural Disorders: Clinical Descriptions and Diagnostic Guidelines*. World Health Organization, Geneva.

Wu, P., Hoven, C.W., Cohen, P., Liu, X., Moore, R.E., Tiet, Q., Okezie, N., Wicks, J., and Bird, H.R. (2001). Factors associated with use of mental health services for depression by children and adolescents. *Psychiatric Services*, **52**, 189–195.

Zoccolillo, M. (1992). Co-occurrence of conduct disorder and its adult outcomes with depressive and anxiety disorders: a review. *Journal of the American Academy of Child and Adolescent Psychiatry*, **31**, 547–556.

Chapter 5

Early adult life

Peter M. Lewinsohn and John R. Seeley

While it is clear from the previous chapters that childhood and adolescent depression commonly occurs, we know little about the continuity of such conditions into adulthood. Hammen and Garber (2001) recently noted that investigators of youth and adult depression have pursued separate tasks for the most part. That is, both fields of research have largely centered on cross-sectional or short-term longitudinal studies, with little focus on bridging the transitional period between childhood and adulthood. As a result, most approaches to the lifespan perspective have been based on disjointed, developmentally specific investigations rather than being based on longitudinal studies that span across developmental periods. According to a report by the Institute of Medicine (IOM; Mrazek and Haggerty, 1994: 116), 'The transition to adulthood is poorly understood in spite of the fact that it is probably the age period when most adult disorders have their peak rates of incidence'. The IOM report further states (p. 117), 'Prospective epidemiological studies that estimate incidence of specific risk factors and disorders in childhood, adolescence, and during the transition to adulthood, from age fifteen to twenty-five, are greatly needed for prevention research. Such studies should help in clarifying the mechanisms linking risk factors to the first occurrence of disorder'. Indeed, a report by the National Institute of Mental Health Workgroup on the Development and Natural History of Mood Disorders (Costello *et al.*, 2001) recently restated these concerns.

It is well established that major depressive disorder (MDD) occurs in older adolescents at levels comparable to adults, with point prevalence estimated at 3–8 per cent (e.g. Kashani *et al.*, 1987; Velez *et al.*, 1989; Fleming and Offord, 1990; McGee *et al.*, 1990; Lewinsohn *et al.*, 1993; Birmaher *et al.*, 1996; Verhulst *et al.*, 1997). In light of its high prevalence, it is important to examine the course and outcome of MDD in youth. Although several longitudinal projects with children and adolescents have been conducted, only a few have followed research participants into adulthood (Garber *et al.*, 1988; Harrington *et al.*, 1990; Rao *et al.*, 1995; Pine *et al.*, 1998; Reinherz *et al.*, 1999a; Weissman *et al.*, 1999). As a result, less is known about the long-term course of child and adolescent MDD and its continuity with adult MDD. In general, these studies indicate that while most adolescents recover from the index MDD episode, the risk of recurrence in young adulthood is substantial. In the three studies that used comparison groups, the rate of mood disorders in adulthood was significantly higher among children and adolescents with MDD than children and adolescents with non-affective disorders (Garber *et al.*, 1988; Harrington *et al.*, 1990) and normal controls (Rao *et al.*, 1995). By contrast, depressed youth did not differ from psychiatric controls on rates of non-affective disorders in adulthood (Garber *et al.*, 1988; Harrington *et al.*, 1990), although the rate of anxiety disorders in adulthood among depressed youth was higher than among normal children and adolescents (Rao *et al.*, 1995). Furthermore, most of the previous studies following depressed youth into adulthood have used relatively small samples of cases from clinical settings. Whereas most children and adolescents with MDD do not seek treatment (e.g. Offord *et al.*, 1987; Keller *et al.*, 1991; Lewinsohn *et al.*, 1998), and treated samples of children and adolescents are biased in a number of respects (Goodman *et al.*, 1997), the importance of longitudinal studies of community samples cannot be overemphasized.

In this chapter, we describe a program of research on depression among adolescents followed into young adulthood that has been conducted since the mid-1980s at the Oregon Research Institute, in Eugene, Oregon, US. Our data set puts us in a unique position to address several issues regarding the transition to adulthood such as (a) the continuity of depression and other psychopathology from adolescence to early adulthood, (b) risk factors for first onset and recurrent depression during young adulthood, and (c) psychosocial functioning during young adulthood of those who experienced an episode of depression during childhood or adolescence. Lastly, some clinical implications for intervention and directions for future research are discussed.

The Oregon adolescent depression project

In 1987 we began a large, prospective, epidemiologic study on adolescent depression as well as other mental disorders, entitled the Oregon Adolescent Depression Project (OADP). Participants were randomly selected in three cohorts from nine senior high schools representative of urban and rural districts in western Oregon. Sampling was proportional to size of the school, grade within school, and gender within grade. A total of 1709 adolescents completed the initial assessment (T_1) which included a diagnostic interview and a questionnaire assessment. Approximately one year later (T_2), 1507 (88 per cent) of the participants returned for a second diagnostic interview and questionnaire assessment. Participants were assessed on a comprehensive array of psychosocial constructs either known to be associated with depression in adults or hypothesized to be important with respect to depression in adolescents. We recently completed a third diagnostic assessment (T_3) with a randomly selected subset of OADP participants $(n = 941)$ near the time of their twenty-fourth birthday and are currently in the process of collecting a fourth diagnostic assessment (T_4) from the participants around their thirtieth birthday. In addition, a family history study of the first-degree relatives $(n = 2750)$ of the OADP probands was conducted near the time of the T_3 assessment which provides data on the rates of psychopathology in parents and siblings.

Average age of the OADP sample at T_1 was 16.6 (SD = 1.2, range = 14–18). Slightly over half of the participants (53 per cent) were female; 91 per cent were White; 12 per cent had repeated a grade in school; and 53 per cent were living with both biological parents at the time of the T_1 interview. Most participants resided in households in which one or both parents worked as a minor professional or professional (for more detail, see Lewinsohn et al., 1993). All probands with a history of MDD at T_2 $(n = 360)$ or a history of non-mood disorders $(n = 284)$, and approximately half of adolescents with no history of psychopathology by T_2 were randomly selected $(n = 457)$ and were invited to participate in a T_3 evaluation. Of the 1101 T_2 participants selected for a T_3 interview, 941 (85 per cent) completed the T_3 assessment. The mean time between the T_2 and T_3 assessments was 6.8 years (SD = 1.4). Women were more likely than men to complete the T_3 assessments (88.9 per cent vs 81.0 per cent); χ^2 (1, $n = 1101$) = 13.55, $p < 0.001$. However, there were no significant differences in T_3 participation as a function of other demographics or T_2 diagnostic status.

Between 1995 and 1998 we recruited and diagnostically interviewed the first-degree relatives (parents and siblings 14 years of age and older) of the T_3 OADP participants for lifetime psychopathology. To supplement the direct interviews and ensure that at least some data were available even for relatives who could not be directly interviewed, informant data on first-degree relatives were collected from probands or another relative. Efforts were made to (a) conduct direct interviews with all living first-degree relatives, (b) obtain family history information on each relative from at least one informant (generally the proband), and (c) obtain two sources of data for all relatives. Of the 941 probands with T_3 data, family diagnostic data were available for 802 (85 per cent). Family diagnostic information was obtained for an additional thirty-eight probands who were selected for the T_3 interview but declined participation. Therefore, family diagnostic information was available for a total of 840 families of T_2 participants, which consisted of the 2750 first-degree relatives. Direct interviews were conducted with 1744 (63.4 per cent) relatives and at least two sources of data were available for 2310 (84.0 per cent) of the family members.

Proband diagnostic information regarding current and past disorders as per the Diagnostic and Statistical Manual of Mental Disorders (DSM-III-R; American Psychiatric Association, 1987; DSM-IV; American Psychiatric Association, 1994) was collected using adolescent report on the Schedule for Affective Disorders and Schizophrenia for School-Age Children (K-SADS; Orvaschel *et al.*, 1982) at point of entry into study, and in conjunction with the Longitudinal Interval Follow-up Evaluation (LIFE; Keller *et al.*, 1987) at subsequent observation points. Parents and siblings were interviewed using either the Structured Clinical Interview for DSM-III-R, non-patient version (SCID-NP) or the K-SADS employed in the T_1 proband assessment, modified for collection of DSM-IV criteria. Family history data were collected using the revised Family Informant Schedule and Criteria (FISC; Mannuzza and Fyer, 1990), based on the Family History Research Diagnostic Criteria (FH-RDC) modified for DSM-IV criteria. Best-estimate diagnoses were derived, blind to proband diagnoses, for relatives using all available data by the four senior diagnosticians on the project. Most diagnostic interviewers had an advanced degree in clinical or counseling psychology or social work, and all were extensively trained prior to data collection. Inter-rater reliability of the interviews was high and comparable to what has been found in other studies (e.g. kappas generally greater than 0.80).

Continuity of depression and other psychopathology from adolescence to early adulthood

In this section, we summarize OADP research findings (Lewinsohn *et al.*, 1999*b*) that examine whether youths with a history of MDD are at increased risk for new episodes of MDD in adulthood, and whether they are at increased risk for other affective and non-affective disorders as adults. Participants with a history of MDD in childhood or adolescence were compared to (a) participants with a history of adjustment disorder with depressed mood prior to age nineteen (which may be considered to be a milder form of depression), (b) participants with other non-affective disorders prior to age nineteen (primarily anxiety, substance use, and disruptive behaviour disorders), and (c) participants with no history of any psychiatric disorder prior to age nineteen.

The rates of psychiatric disorders from nineteen to twenty-three years of age as a function of diagnostic status through age eighteen are presented in Table 5.1. As can be seen, 45 per cent of the adolescent MDD group experienced a recurrence of MDD between ages nineteen and twenty-three, compared to MDD first incidence rates of 34 per cent in the adolescent adjustment disorder group, 28 per cent in the adolescent non-affective group, and 19 per cent in the adolescent no disorder group. Four additional participants in the adolescent MDD group (1.7 per cent), and no participant in the remaining adolescent diagnostic groups, developed dysthymia in this time period. Six participants (0.8 per cent) were diagnosed with bipolar disorder between nineteen and twenty-three years of age (three from the adolescent MDD group, two from the adolescent non-affective disorder group, and one from the adolescent no disorder group).

The rates of psychiatric disorders in young adulthood were compared with three planned contrasts: (1) adolescent MDD vs no disorder, (2) adolescent MDD vs non-affective disorder, and (3) adolescent MDD vs adjustment disorder. Group differences were evaluated using hierarchical multiple logistic regression analyses, with gender, household composition, and maximum parental education at T_1 entered as the first block, followed by adolescent diagnostic group status with the three contrasts entered as the second block, and interactions between demographic variables and adolescent diagnostic group status entered as the third block. Given a significant contrast in the second block, the odds ratio (OR; adjusted for demographic characteristics, with 95 per cent confidence interval [CI]) for increased risk in the adolescent MDD group was calculated and appears in the last three columns of Table 5.1.

As can be seen, compared to adolescents without a history of psychopathology, participants with adolescent MDD had significantly higher rates of future MDD, non-affective Axis I disorders, and any Axis I disorder in young adulthood, as well as elevated scores on the antisocial and borderline personality disorder dimensions. The difference between adolescent MDD and no disorder groups in rates of future non-affective disorder appeared to be due to the presence of another mental disorder in the individuals with adolescent MDD; when the rate of non-affective disorder from nineteen to twenty-three years was examined for the no disorder group vs individuals with 'pure' (non-comorbid) adolescent MDD, differences were non-significant (19.5 per cent vs 26.6 per cent, respectively).

Table 5.1 Frequency of diagnosis in young adulthood as a function of adolescent diagnostic group

Diagnosis 19–23		Adolescent diagnostic group				Adjusted[1] OR (95% CI)		
		MDD	ADJUST	NONAFF	ND	MDD vs ND	MDD vs NONAFF	MDD vs ADJUST
MDD	n	107/238	25/73	37/131	50/271	3.2 (2.2–4.9)	1.8 (1.2–3.0)	ns
	%	45.0	34.2	28.2	18.5			
ADJUST	n	22/261	3/71	14/133	22/272	ns	ns	ns
	%	8.4	4.2	10.5	8.1			
NONAFF	n	72/217	20/65	30/83	53/272	2.3 (1.5–3.6)	ns	ns
	%	33.2	30.8	36.1	19.5			
Any Axis I	n	124/199	30/63	45/83	102/272	2.7 (1.8–3.9)	ns	1.8 (1.01–3.2)
	%	62.3	47.6	54.2	37.5			
Axis II	n	7/261	1/73	3/133	2/272	ns	ns	ns
	%	2.7	1.4	2.3	0.7			
Antisocial PDE score	n	25/255	2/65	22/128	8/266	6.1 (2.6–14.5)	ns	4.7 (1.04–21.1)
	%	9.8	3.1	17.2	3.0			
Borderline PDE score	n	25/255	2/65	6/128	2/266	14.9 (3.4–64.8)	ns	ns
	%	9.8	3.1	4.7	0.8			

Note:

[1] Adjusted for gender, family structure, and parental education at T1

MDD = major depressive disorder; ND = no disorder; NONAFF = non-affective disorder; ADJUST = adjustment disorder with depressed mood; PD = Personality disorder examination; OR = odds ratio; CI = confidence interval; ns = not significant. Twenty-five participants had missing PDE scores

Compared to the adolescent non-affective participants, adolescent MDD increased the probability for future MDD. The lack of a significant difference between the adolescent MDD and non-affective groups on rates of future non-affective disorder was not due to the inclusion of adolescent MDD cases who had another mental disorder; individuals with 'pure' adolescent MDD were compared to participants in the adolescent non-affective group and did not differ in rates of future non-affective disorder (26.6 per cent vs 36.1 per cent).

Although they were not significantly elevated on rates of future MDD or non-affective disorder, compared to participants with adolescent adjustment disorder, individuals with adolescent MDD were significantly more likely to develop an Axis I disorder in young adulthood and to be elevated on the antisocial personality dimensional score.

Additional analyses examined differences in the occurrence of future MDD and non-affective disorders among the three diagnostic groups who had not experienced adolescent MDD: adolescent non-affective and adjustment disorder groups did not differ from each other and were both significantly elevated compared to those without a history of psychopathology (MDD incidence: adolescent adjustment vs no disorder adjusted OR = 2.11 [95 per cent CI = 1.18–3.76]; adjustment vs non-affective adjusted OR = 1.71 [95 per cent CI = 1.05–2.81]; non-affective disorder incidence: adolescent adjustment vs no disorder adjusted OR = 20.6 [95 per cent CI = 1.11–3.82]; adjustment vs non-affective adjusted OR = 2.34 [95 per cent CI = 1.36–4.04]).

The results clearly illustrate a strong pattern of continuity for depression, in that the rate of MDD in young adulthood was significantly elevated in the adolescent MDD group. To wit, 45 per cent of adolescents with a history of MDD developed a new episode of MDD for the 19–23 age period, which translates into an average annual MDD recurrence rate of 9 per cent over the 5-year period. Annual MDD incidence rates for the non-affective and no disorder groups were significantly lower (5.6 per cent and 3.7 per cent, respectively).

Those with adolescent MDD also had elevated rates of non-affective disorders between the nineteen and twenty-three age period. However, rates of future non-affective disorder among the adolescent MDD participants did not differ from rates among adolescents with non-affective disorders. These results are consistent with previous studies using clinical samples in finding a higher rate of non-affective disorders in young adulthood among depressed children and adolescents than normal controls (Rao *et al.*, 1995), but a similar rate compared to children and adolescents with non-affective disorders (Garber *et al.*, 1988; Harrington *et al.*, 1990).

Adolescents with MDD also exhibited elevated rates of antisocial and borderline personality disorder traits, which is consistent with previous findings of early onset depression being associated with higher rates of various personality disorders (Fava *et al.*, 1996; Cohen *et al.*, 1998).

An interesting feature of this study was the inclusion of a near-neighbour comparison group of adolescents with adjustment disorder with depressed mood. The results suggest that the prognosis of adolescent adjustment disorder is nearly as bad as adolescent MDD, in that rates of future MDD and non-affective disorder for the adolescent adjustment disorder and the adolescent MDD groups did not differ. Thus, the present results are somewhat at variance with the finding of Kovacs *et al.* (1984) that child/adolescent patients with MDD were at greater risk of subsequent MDD compared to patients with adjustment disorder. However, when all Axis I disorders developing during the 19–23 age period were combined into a single category, the adolescent MDD group had an elevated incidence of disorder relative to the adolescent adjustment disorder group.

It was also interesting to note that adjustment disorder during adolescence was not associated with significantly elevated rates of adjustment disorder during young adulthood. The absence of diagnostic continuity for adjustment disorder may relate to the fortuitous nature of stressful life events that precipitate this disorder. Nonetheless, individuals who succumb to adjustment disorder with depressed mood in the face of a stressor as adolescents are at elevated risk for future MDD as young adults.

Among adolescents with MDD, the presence of a comorbid non-affective disorder increased the probability of future non-affective psychopathology (both Axis I and II). Regarding the potential impact of comorbid dysthymia, almost all of the adolescents with lifetime MDD and dysthymia also had a non-affective disorder, and once the effects of non-affective disorder were taken into consideration, the presence of dysthymia was not uniquely associated with increased risk of future psychopathology among the MDD adolescents.

Gender effects in this study were few. In general, females were more likely to develop MDD and adjustment disorder in young adulthood, while males were more likely to develop non-affective Axis I disorders and Axis II psychopathology. However, gender did not significantly interact with adolescent diagnostic group in predicting psychopathology in young adulthood. Previous studies have been inconsistent regarding whether women with MDD are at greater risk for recurrence than men (Amenson and Lewinsohn, 1981; Kessler *et al.*, 1993; Lewinsohn *et al.*, 2001a) and this issue deserves continued attention.

In addition to examining the continuity of MDD to early adulthood, we also examined the continuity of suicidal behaviour (Lewinsohn *et al.*, 2001b).

Period prevalence rates of suicide attempt were examined in three developmental periods (a) childhood, defined as ages 5–11, (b) adolescence, defined as ages 12–18, and (c) young adulthood, defined as ages 19–23. The percentage of female and male participants who had made a suicide attempt (first or recurrent) in each of the three time periods was contrasted, with results shown in Table 5.2. Even though five of the six children who made an attempt in the 5–11 year group were girls, this difference was not statistically significant. In adolescence, female participants had a significantly higher rate of suicide attempts, compared to male participants. However, the gender difference did not attain statistical significance during young adulthood.

For comparative purposes, also shown in Table 5.2 are the percentage of male and female participants who experienced an episode of MDD (first

Table 5.2 Gender differences in suicide attempt and major depressive disorder during childhood, adolescence, and young adulthood

Outcome time period	Female sample	Male sample	Chi-square	OR (95% CI)
Suicide attempt (%)				
5–11 years of age				
Observed[1]	0.9	0.2	1.88	3.78 (0.43–32.26)
Weighted[2]	0.8	0.2	3.12	5.03 (0.60–41.98)
12–18 years of age				
Observed	12.8	6.0	12.70***	2.31 (1.43–3.75)
Weighted	9.9	4.2	16.68***	2.53 (1.58–4.04)
19–23 years of age				
Observed	3.7	2.5	1.12	1.51 (0.70–3.26)
Weighted	3.2	1.8	2.44	1.77 (0.86–3.67)
Occurrence of MDD (%)				
5–11 years of age				
Observed	6.9	1.7	15.22***	4.16 (1.83–9.43)
Weighted	5.1	1.2	17.97***	4.61 (2.04–10.41)
12–18 years of age				
Observed	40.1	21.1	39.00***	2.49 (1.86–3.35)
Weighted	30.2	14.8	44.95***	2.49 (1.89–3.29)
19–23 years of age				
Observed	36.5	19.7	32.64***	2.36 (1.74–3.19)
Weighted	33.8	16.9	50.03***	2.51 (1.93–3.27)

[1] Discriminant function = 1, $N = 941$

[2] Discriminant function = 1, $N = 1320$

***$p < 0.001$

or recurrent) during the three developmental periods. Significant gender differences in MDD occurrence were present for all three periods, with female participants having consistently higher rates than male participants. Several somewhat unexpected findings are noteworthy. First, without disaggregating results for male and female participants, we would have erroneously concluded that the suicide attempt rate decreases from adolescence to young adulthood. In fact, a significant drop in prevalence rate is only evident for young women. Future research needs to examine if prevalence rates remain at this low level as the participants move further into adulthood.

Disappearance of the gender difference for suicide attempts by young adulthood is not accounted for by a parallel decrease in the gender difference for MDD. Female gender is significantly associated with MDD in each of the three developmental periods, with an odds ratio greater than two in each time period. Research to identify factors that account for the high rate of depression in females beginning at a very early age deserves a high priority. Similarly, research to explain the high rate of suicide attempt in female adolescents and the decline in the suicide attempt rate in young female adults is needed.

Risk factors for first onset and recurrent depression during young adulthood

Results of recent studies (Post *et al.*, 1994; Lewinsohn *et al.*, 1999a) have suggested that the risk factors for first episode may be different from those that predict depression recurrence or persistence (Warner *et al.*, 1992; Goodyer *et al.*, 1997; Ilardi *et al.*, 1997). As we have reported in the previous section, given that there is a high rate of first incidence and recurrence of MDD in young adulthood, this period of the lifespan provides a unique opportunity to examine the risk factors for first and recurrent episodes. Thus, the question that we address in this section is: What putative risk factors for depression assessed during adolescence predict first incident and/or recurrent MDD during young adulthood? The risk factors are based on an extensive battery of psychosocial measures administered at the T_1 assessment (mean age = 16.6) that were chosen for inclusion because they had been shown or were hypothesized to be related to depression during adolescence. Details regarding the measures and their psychometric properties have been reported previously (Lewinsohn *et al.*, 1994). Comorbid adolescent psychopathology (lifetime history at T_1) is also included in the set of risk factors. In addition, traits measuring antisocial and personality disorders which we assessed during young adulthood are also included. We also included two measures regarding family psychopathology: (a) the proportion of first-degree relatives who had history of MDD, and (b) the proportion of first-degree relatives who had a history of non-mood disorders. Lastly, consistent with the expectation that having experienced an episode of depression creates vulnerabilities which affect recurrence, clinical aspects of the adolescent MDD episode (e.g. early onset, longer duration, recurrence during adolescence, greater severity, treatment utilization, and suicide attempts) were also examined as predictors of recurrence during young adulthood.

To compare the OADP risk factors of MDD onset vs recurrence in young adulthood (age 19–23 years), two sets of analyses were performed. The first set was restricted to adolescents who did not have a history of MDD by age eighteen and were followed to age twenty-four ($n = 605$); those who developed MDD during young adulthood ($n = 141$) were compared to those who did not develop MDD ($n = 464$) on the set of predictor variables. The second set were restricted to adolescents who had a history of MDD by age eighteen and were followed to age twenty-four ($n = 274$); those who developed a recurrent episode of MDD ($n = 125$) were compared to those who did not experience MDD recurrence ($n = 149$) on the same set of adolescent predictors. The first set of analyses is presented here for the first time whereas the second set has been previously reported in Lewinsohn et al. (2000). For each predictor, logistic regression analysis was used to calculate the odds ratio for first onset MDD episodes and recurrent MDD episodes. In addition, potential moderating effects of sex were also tested with interaction terms in the logistic regression analyses. The significant bivariate associations are summarized in Table 5.3. Of the twenty-eight putative risk factors of first onset, sixteen (54 per cent) were significant predictors (at $p < 0.05$). Of the thirty-four putative risk factors of recurrence, only eight (24 per cent) significantly predicted MDD recurrence during young adulthood. The only significant interaction with sex was obtained for conflict with parents predicting MDD recurrence; the association was significant for female participants but not for male participants.

To examine whether the variables distinguishing the MDD outcomes remained significant when controlling for the effects of the other variables, summary multiple logistic regression (MLR) analyses were conducted using the likelihood-ratio backward selection procedure for each set of bivariate predictors. Given the stronger associations obtained for recurrent MDD in the family members compared to any MDD in the family members, the former was used in MLR analyses. The variables with unique and independent effects retained in the final model for each column are indicated in Table 5.3 with an asterisk. Regarding the first incidence MLR, four variables were retained in the final solution: female gender, daily hassles, poor physical health, and proportion of family members with recurrent MDD. Using

Table 5.3 Adolescent predictors of MDD in young adulthood: first onset vs recurrence

Adolescent predictor	Young adult MDD	
	First onset OR (95% CI)	Recurrence OR (95% CI)
Demographic		
Sex (female)	2.03* (1.38–2.98)	2.29 (1.33–3.95)*
Race/ethnicity	ns	ns
Family intactness	ns	ns
Parental education	ns	ns
Psychosocial		
Depression symptom level	1.36 (1.14–1.63)	ns
Negative cognitions	ns	ns
Attributional style	ns	ns
Self-esteem	1.32 (1.09–1.59)	ns
Excessive emotional reliance on others	1.26 (1.05–1.52)	1.31 (1.03–1.67)
Self-perceived social competence	ns	ns
Coping skills	1.27 (1.05–1.54)	ns
Social support: friends	ns	ns
Social support: family	ns	ns
Conflict with parents	1.22 (1.01–1.46)	1.38 (1.01–1.87)*[1]
Daily hassles	1.39* (1.16–1.68)	ns
Major life events	ns	ns
Academic problems	1.21 (1.01–1.46)	ns
Physical health	1.49* (1.24–1.78)	ns
Other psychopathology		
Dysthymia	3.93 (1.40–11.03)	ns
Anxiety disorders	1.86 (1.08–3.21)	ns
Substance abuse/dependence	1.66 (1.07–2.56)	ns
Daily cigarette use	1.87 (1.12–3.14)	ns
CD/ODD	ns	ns
Axis II psychopathology		
PDE antisocial	ns	ns
PDE borderline	5.34 (1.87–15.29)	1.80* (1.42–2.28)
Family history of psychopathology		
MDD 2.10 (1.01–4.36)	3.59 (1.50–8.63)	
Recurrent MDD	4.19* (1.68–10.43)	9.46* (2.92–30.61)
Non-mood disorder	ns	ns
Characteristics of adolescent MDD episodes		
Age of onset (<13 vs 14+)	na	ns

Table 5.3 *(continued)*

Adolescent predictor	Young adult MDD	
	First onset OR (95% CI)	Recurrence OR (95% CI)
Duration of first episode (2–8 vs 9+)	na	1.81 (1.08–3.03)
Single vs. recurrent episode	na	3.20* (1.54–6.65)
Severity of worst episode	na	ns
Treatment utilization	na	ns
History of suicide attempt	na	ns

Notes:

[1] Significant only for female participants; association is presented for the female sample

* Variable retained in multiple logistic regression final solution

MDD = major depressive disorder; CD/ODD =conduct disorder/oppositional defiant disorder; PDE = personality disorder examination; OR = odds ratio; CI = confidence interval; ns = non-significant; na = not applicable

the prior probability of group membership (i.e. Bayes' rule), the final solution correctly classified 66 per cent of the participants (specificity and sensitivity = 66 per cent).

With respect to the MLR final solution for recurrent MDD, the following predictors were retained in the model: female gender, multiple MDD episodes in adolescence, proportion of family members with recurrent MDD, borderline personality disorder symptoms, and the interaction of conflict with parents by sex (indicating a significant association for females but not for males). The solution correctly classified 72 per cent of the participants (sensitivity = 73 per cent; specificity = 72 per cent).

There are several noteworthy findings from these analyses. First, there were more than twice as many significant predictors for first onset than for recurrence. In part, this finding may have been impacted by having a larger reference sample for the first onset than for recurrence (605 vs 274). However, there was adequate power (>0.80) for the recurrence analysis to predict moderately small effects (Cohen's w = 0.20). Despite having more significant bivariate predictors, the summary MLR model for MDD onset retained only four variables and did not correctly classify as many participants as did the five variables retained in the summary MLR model for MDD recurrence (66 per cent vs 72 per cent). Thus, although the number of significant predictors differed between first onset and recurrence, the multivariate predictive ability was comparable.

Most of the psychosocial variables that predicted MDD onset in young adulthood have been previously shown to predict MDD during adolescence

(Lewinsohn *et al.*, 1994). Of the few that did not predict during young adulthood (i.e. family intactness, negative cognitions, attributional style, social support, and major life events), the most plausible explanations for these non-significant findings are (a) that their prognostic impact in previous studies is time-limited, or (b) that they are specific to adolescent depression. Thus, the extent to which a variable's predictive ability diminishes as a function of time, and the specificity of risk factors for adolescent vs adult depression, needs to be explored in future research.

The majority of psychosocial variables assessed during adolescence were not found to predict recurrence of MDD, with the exception of excessive emotional reliance and conflict with parents (for female participants only). Excessive emotional reliance on others is a component of the broader construct of interpersonal dependency (Hirschfeld *et al.*, 1989) and has been implicated theoretically in the etiology of depression, especially in the psychoanalytic literature (e.g. Hirschfeld *et al.*, 1976; Blatt *et al.*, 1982). Emotional reliance was assessed using the Emotional Reliance Scale of the Interpersonal Dependency Inventory (Hirschfeld *et al.*, 1977) and refers to an excessive desire for support and approval from others, anxiety when left alone or when considered abandoned, and interpersonal sensitivity. We previously reported that excessive emotional reliance predicted depression onset in adolescents (Lewinsohn *et al.*, 1994) and that it remained elevated after MDD recovery (Rohde *et al.*, 1994). The present results indicate that emotional reliance is also predictive of the MDD onset and recurrence in young adulthood, underscoring its centrality to depression theory. Interestingly, conflict with parents also emerged as a risk factor for MDD recurrence for female participants only. As with excessive emotional reliance, a conflictual relationship with parents is of an interpersonal nature and may be a persistent problem for depressed adolescents. Taken together, these findings provide support to the interpersonal approach to depression (Weissman and Paykel, 1974; Youngren and Lewinsohn, 1980; Coyne *et al.*, 1991; Hammen, 1999).

There was no evidence that adolescent comorbidity acted as a risk factor for recurrent MDD in young adulthood. Contrary to previous research (e.g. Kovacs *et al.*, 1984; Warner *et al.*, 1992), comorbid dysthymia in the present study failed to predict MDD recurrence. Unlike previous research on the impact of double depression (i.e. MDD superimposed on a preexisting dysthymia), adolescent MDD and dysthymia in the present study occurred largely at different periods. Future research needs to disentangle whether concurrent comorbidity of MDD and dysthymia specifically confers a risk for MDD recurrence.

With respect to Axis II psychopathology, borderline traits were found to be associated with both MDD onset and recurrence in young adulthood.

Several adult studies have suggested strong comorbidity between depression and borderline personality disorder and symptomatology (e.g. Akiskal *et al.*, 1983; Farmer and Nelson-Gray, 1990; Oldham *et al.*, 1995; Skodol *et al.*, 1999). The present findings on Axis II psychopathology need to be qualified in two respects. First, rates of personality disorders were low, so elevated dimensional scores were generally in the subthreshold range. Second, the Axis II data were obtained at T_3. Therefore, the direction of these associations cannot be determined.

The proportion of family members with MDD (particularly recurrent MDD) predicted MDD onset and recurrence in young adulthood. These findings are consistent with previous research indicating that the presence of MDD in family members significantly increases the likelihood of MDD recurrence in adults (e.g. Gonzales *et al.*, 1985; Bland *et al.*, 1986; Merikangas *et al.*, 1994). Furthermore, based on the magnitude of the associations, recurrent familial MDD appears to have a stronger liability than non-recurrent familial MDD.

Risk processes for first vs recurrent MDD episodes

In addition to identifying differences between the predictors of first onset vs recurrence, it is important to consider how the risk processes may differ. Such processes include mediation and moderation between environmental influences, vulnerabilities, and protective factors. Recent theories of depression suggest that different risk mechanisms or processes may be implicated in first vs subsequent episodes of MDD. For example, Post (1992, Post *et al.*, 1996) proposed a 'kindling' or 'stress sensitization' model in which a higher level of stress is required to trigger an initial episode of MDD, but that increasingly lower levels of stress are required for subsequent episodes, and eventually episodes occur in the absence of discernible stressors. Although there have been some negative findings, and most of the studies testing this hypothesis have been retrospective, a number of studies have reported that stress is more strongly associated with first MDD episodes than with recurrences (Post, 1992). Similarly, Teasdale (1983, 1988) has hypothesized that vulnerability to severe depressive states is influenced by patterns of information processing that occur during mild states of dysphoria. He emphasized the importance of differentiating between first onsets and recurrent episodes of depression, and proposed that the links between depressogenic information-processing styles and dysphoric affect will be stronger among individuals who have previously experienced a depressive episode than among previously non-depressed persons. Teasdale's theory has been supported by a number of studies finding that individuals with a history of previous MDD episodes are more prone to exhibit depressogenic cognitions than never-depressed individuals following a dysphoric mood induction procedure (Teasdale and Dent, 1987; Miranda and Persons, 1988; Miranda *et al.*, 1990).

Our previous research (Lewinsohn *et al.*, 1999*a*) was the first to prospectively compare the roles of depressive symptoms, dysfunctional thinking, and stress in the development of first onsets and recurrences of depression in adolescents. Our results were consistent with both Post's (1992) and Teasdale's (1983, 1988) models, suggesting that stress plays a greater role in first episodes of MDD, while the combination of dysphoric mood and dysfunctional thinking play a greater role in recurrent episodes. In another study, we also examined the risk conferred by a recent romantic break-up as a predictor of first onset vs recurrence of MDD during adolescence (Monroe *et al.*, 1999). Consistent with Post's theory, a recent break-up predicted the first onset of MDD during the ensuing 12 months but did not predict MDD recurrence.

Given that the models developed by Post and Teasdale were based on theories regarding depression in adults, the confirmation of these hypotheses with OADP adolescents suggests that similar processes appear to be involved in first vs recurrent episodes for both adolescents and adults. Furthermore, the degree of overlap between the OADP risk factors for adolescent-onset (Lewinsohn *et al.*, 1994) and those for young adult-onset described previously in this chapter suggests that similar processes may be involved for the onset of MDD in adolescence and young adulthood.

Psychosocial functioning during young adulthood

A growing literature documents the serious negative associations between MDD and the functioning of adolescents and adults. Researchers have found depression to be related to difficulties in academic and occupational performance (e.g. Kessler and Frank, 1996; Winokur and Tsuang, 1996); interpersonal conflict and relationship discord (Kandel and Davies, 1986; Garber *et al.*, 1988; Kessler *et al.*, 1998); early childbearing (Rao *et al.*, 1995; Bardone *et al.*, 1996; Kessler *et al.*, 1997), increased levels of stress (e.g. Hammen, 1991), as well as increased physical health problems and treatment utilization (e.g. Kandel and Davies, 1986).

In this section, we summarize OADP findings on the psychosocial functioning of young adults who have experienced an episode of MDD during childhood/adolescence (Lewinsohn *et al.*, 2001*c*). These data allow us to address three issues: (1) To what extent is the psychosocial functioning of young adults who experienced an episode of MDD during adolescence impaired relative to those who did not experience adolescent MDD? (2) To what extent are the impairments evident only in those with comorbid non-mood disorders? (3) Are the impairments in young adult functioning detectable even in formerly depressed adolescents who remain free of MDD in young adulthood?

Young adult psychosocial functioning in the present study is broadly defined to include measures of academic and occupational performance, marital and parenting status, social support, stress, life satisfaction, mental health utilization, physical health, and regular cigarette smoking. Based on previous research, we expected that, compared to their never-depressed counterparts, the formerly depressed individuals would show lower educational and occupational achievement, higher rates of early childbearing, higher rates of divorce and separation, elevated levels of minor hassles and major life events, lower levels of life satisfaction and social support, more frequent treatment utilization, poorer physical health, and higher rates of cigarette smoking.

As is now well known, many depressed adolescents and adults have comorbid mental disorders (e.g. Rohde *et al.*, 1991; Kessler, 1997). Therefore, our second issue involves the impact of a comorbid adolescent psychopathology on measures of psychosocial functioning. It is important to examine the degree to which the measures of psychosocial functioning we expect to find in formerly depressed young adults are dependent upon the experience of a comorbid mental disorder. Harrington *et al.* (1991) compared the adult outcomes of depressed child/adolescent patients with and without conduct disorder and found that depressed children with conduct disorder had poorer short-term outcome (less recovery and a greater degree of handicap at discharge) and a greater likelihood of adult criminality. Although not statistically significant, differences in almost all assessed domains of adult social functioning (e.g. work, intimate relationships, friendships) suggested that children with comorbid depression/conduct disorder tended to be more impaired than were depressed children without conduct disorder. Our expectation is that depressed adolescents with comorbid disorders would show higher rates of measures of psychosocial functioning than would those with pure adolescent depression in several areas of functioning.

The third issue is whether these impairments are found even in formerly depressed adolescents who have not experienced another episode of depression or another mental disorder as adults. Being depressed during adolescence is a powerful predictor of developing depression and/or other mental disorders in young adulthood (Lewinsohn *et al.*, 1999b) and it is possible that the occurrence of MDD and other psychopathology during young adulthood is what accounts for any measures of psychosocial functioning that are found to be associated with adolescent MDD. Geller *et al.* (2001) compared the psychosocial functioning in young adulthood of former child patients with prepubertal MDD to a normal comparison group. A number of impairments were identified (e.g. relationship difficulties with parents, siblings, and friends; functioning problems in household, school, and work; lower quality of life and social adjustment ratings), but these differences became non-significant when results were restricted to the formerly depressed patients who had not experienced recurrent mood disorders or substance use disorders in the past five years. Our expectation is that participants with recurrent MDD and participants who experience other mental disorders during young adulthood will account for the majority of measures of psychosocial functioning effects, but that even formerly depressed participants who do not experience MDD or additional psychopathology in young adulthood will show some evidence of impairment.

Only three of the measures of young adult functioning examined in the present study were unrelated to adolescent depression: marital status, early divorce/separation, and cohabitation. In a previous paper based on a subset of the OADP sample, Gotlib *et al.* (1998) reported that being married was associated with a history of adolescent MDD for the younger female participants (40 per cent of the 19–23-year-old women with a history of MDD were married vs 29 per cent of same-aged women with no MDD history; $p < 0.05$) but not for the older female participants (38 per cent of 24–26-year-old women with a history of MDD were married vs 45 per cent of same aged women with no MDD history; non-significant difference); marital status was unrelated to MDD history for the male participants. In addition to earlier marriage, a history of adolescent MDD also predicted marital discord for both men and women. Regarding divorce, Kessler *et al.* (1998) found that almost all psychiatric disorders in adults are associated with an increased probability of divorce. Our non-significant findings regarding divorce need to be considered in the context of the relatively young age of our sample (i.e. overall divorce rates were very low). The direction of results in our study suggests that the putative relations between divorce/separation and a history of MDD may become more pronounced at subsequent assessments.

With respect to the second issue, the presence of psychiatric comorbidity with adolescent MDD was most strongly associated with failure to obtain a college degree. Indeed, 'purely' depressed adolescents were more than twice as likely as comorbid depressed adolescents to obtain a college degree (30 per cent vs 14 per cent). Although this was the only comparison that reached the requisite statistical significance level, it is noteworthy that with the single exception of life satisfaction, relative to the pure adolescent MDD group, the adolescent comorbid group exhibited poorer functioning in young adulthood on every measure examined in this study.

As predicted, the psychosocial impairments associated with adolescent MDD were detectable even in participants who remained free of MDD recurrence in young adulthood. These analyses contrasted participants with adolescent (but not young adult) depression vs those who had never experienced MDD. Controlling for the lifetime presence of non-mood disorder, two psychosocial variables were directly related to adolescent MDD: completing college and reporting low levels of family social support. Smaller social networks and poorer physical health in young adulthood initially appeared to be closely associated with adolescent MDD, but became non-significant after adjusting for lifetime non-mood disorders. Clearly, even formerly depressed adolescents who remain free of subsequent psychopathology appear to show some longstanding impairments. It may be the case that the persistence of impaired psychosocial functioning in these specific domains constitutes part of the vulnerability that increases risk for MDD in the future, and it remains for further research to examine this formulation more explicitly.

The potential for gender to moderate group differences in measures of psychosocial functioning was examined, but none of the interactions was significant. This pattern of results suggests that the associations of adolescent MDD with negative aspects in young adult functioning are equally strong for formerly depressed women and men, and that gender differences on the measures of psychosocial functioning do not account for the elevated rates of depression in women. Tempering these conclusions is the fact that our statistical power to detect gender interactions, especially regarding issues of specificity and comorbidity, may have been somewhat limited. Future research on the impact of specificity and comorbidity should strive to ensure adequate representation of the various disorders in both sexes.

Young adulthood is an important stage in the lifespan. It is the time when individuals make important decisions and choices—about education, occupation, relationships—that greatly influence the rest of their lives. The present results indicate that young adults who have experienced an episode of MDD during adolescence exhibit impairments across numerous domains of socioeconomic and psychosocial functioning. These findings replicate previous results of previous research showing pervasive difficulties in psychosocial functioning associated with depression in young adults, including impairments in the areas of interpersonal relationships, academic achievement and occupational roles, health utilization and cigarette smoking (e.g. Kandel and Davies, 1986; Brook *et al.*, 1996; Rao *et al.*, 1999; Reinherz *et al.*, 1999*b*; Geller *et al.*, 2001).

Clinical implications and directions for future research

Throughout the chapter a number of issues have been highlighted that have implications for intervention and that point to directions for future research. We provide a brief synthesis of these issues here.

Several risk factors were identified for depression in young adulthood (e.g. sex, adolescent MDD, family history of MDD, and social-personal factors such as excessive interpersonal dependence and conflict) based on prospective analyses. This knowledge is the critical point of departure for generating and testing hypotheses about possible mechanisms. It is also needed in order to identify those at elevated risk so they can be targeted for prevention and intervention. As Hammen and Garber (2001) note, the most robust findings to date regarding risk factors for depression are (a) being female, (b) having experienced a previous episode of depression, and (c) having a family history of depression. These risk factors were replicated in the OADP sample of adolescents and young adults. Not only do such findings help to identify individuals who are at greatest risk for future depression, theoretical models should address the mechanisms whereby these factors convey a vulnerability to depression. Furthermore, in contrast to the number of studies on risk factors, little attention has been paid to the protective mechanism for guarding against depression. That is, which factors protect high-risk adolescents against becoming depressed again later in adulthood? Such knowledge is critical for developing preventive interventions for depression.

Future research also needs to be sensitive to the possibility that some of the psychosocial characteristics associated with depression may be concomitants (occur only during the episode, but do not exist before or after the episode, i.e. are state-dependent), scars (psychosocial characteristics that are consequences or residual effects of an episode, i.e. did not exist before the episode) and antecedents (i.e. risk factors which precede the occurrence of depression and which are probably most relevant to etiology). Based on longitudinal studies such as the OADP, the putative early risk and protective factors for youth and young adult depression need to be clearly established in order to refine models of etiology and guide prevention efforts. Factors that contribute to the onset of depression need to be distinguished from those that maintain depression or predict depression recurrence. Furthermore, risk and protective factors that are specific to certain developmental periods, or that are gender-specific, should be determined. We would like to suggest that theoretical formulations of depression should incorporate the complexities that have emerged. Findings from the OADP have provided empirical support for risk mechanisms proposed by others in the literature. For example, specific hypotheses proposed by Post (1992, Post et al., 1996) and Teasdale (1983, 1988) regarding differential risk processes for first onset vs recurrent episodes were supported. In addition, several of the OADP findings provide support for those theorists who have emphasized the interpersonal approach to depression vulnerability (e.g. Weissman et al., 1974; Lewinsohn et al., 1982; Coyne et al., 1991; Hammen, 1999), such as excessive emotional reliance and conflict with parents predicting MDD onset and recurrence in young adulthood, as well as the findings on early marriage and marital discord among those with a history of MDD during adolescence. Although the findings presented here based on the OADP need to be cross-validated, we are beginning to provide empirical support for theories regarding the risk mechanisms. Clearly, there is much more work to be accomplished in this area.

Our results serve to emphasize the importance of efforts to prevent the occurrence of depression during adolescence. Such efforts can be aimed at ameliorating psychosocial risk factors for depression (such as the depressotypic thinking style). With the expectation that this will reduce the incidence of depression, this approach is exemplified by the work of Jaycox et al. (1994). Another approach is to target youth who are at elevated risk for becoming depressed either because they are already mildly depressed and/or because they have a depressed parent. This approach is exemplified by the work of Clarke et al. (1995, 2001). Promising results have been obtained with both of these approaches. Given that the period of greatest risk for the incidence of depression extends into early adulthood, similar prevention efforts should be extended into early adulthood. In addition to targeting a reduction in depression symptoms, the intervention could also be aimed at known risk factors for depression (e.g. interpersonal conflicts, coping and interpersonal skills). Hopefully, research will show that by modifying risk factor status it is possible to impact depression prevalence. Research clearly needs to demonstrate that by modifying the risk factors, the incidence of depression can be reduced. It is our hope that by promoting protective factors and ameliorating risk factors early in the lifespan, the longstanding difficulties associated with adolescent depression may be averted.

Acknowledgement

This research was partially supported by National Institute of Mental Health Grants MH40501 and MH50522.

References

Akiskal, H.S., Hirschfeld, R.M.A., and Yerevanian, B.I. (1983). The relationship of personality to affective disorders. *Archives of General Psychiatry*, **40**, 801–810.

Amenson, C.S. and Lewinsohn, P.M. (1981). An investigation into the observed sex difference in prevalence of unipolar depression. *Journal of Abnormal Psychology*, **90**, 1–13.

American Psychiatric Association (1987). *Diagnostic and Statistical Manual of Mental Disorders, III-R*. Author, Washington, DC.

American Psychiatric Association (1994). *Diagnostic and Statistical Manual of Mental Disorders*. (4th edition). Author, Washington, DC.

Bardone, A.M., Moffitt, T.E., Caspi, A., Dickson, N., and Silva, P.A. (1996). Adult mental health and social outcomes of adolescent girls with depression and conduct disorder. *Development and Psychopathology*, **8**, 811–829.

Birmaher, B., Ryan, N.D., Williamson, D.E., Brent, D.A., and Kaufman, J. (1996). Childhood and adolescent depression: A review of the past 10 years. Part II. *Journal of the American Academy of Child and Adolescent Psychiatry*, **35**, 1575–1583.

Birmaher, B., Ryan, N.D., Williamson, D.E., *et al.* (1996). Childhood and adolescent depression: A review of the past 10 years. Part 1. *Journal of the American Academy of Child and Adolescent Psychiatry*, **35**, 1427–1439.

Bland, R.C., Newman, S.C., and Orn, H. (1986). Recurrent and nonrecurrent depression: A family study. *Archives of General Psychiatry*, **43**, 1085–1089.

Blatt, S., Quinlan, D., Chevron, E., McDonald, C., and Zuroff, D. (1982). Dependency and self-criticism: Psychological dimensions of depression. *Journal of Consulting and Clinical Psychology*, **50**, 113–124.

Brook, J.S., Whiteman, M., Finch, S.J., and Cohen, P. (1996). Young adult drug use and delinquency: Childhood antecedents and adolescent mediators. *Journal of the American Academy of Child and Adolescent Psychiatry*, **35**, 1584–1592.

Clarke, G.N., Hawkins, W., Murphy, M., Sheeber, L.B., Lewinsohn, P.M., and Seeley, J.R. (1995). Targeted prevention of unipolar depressive disorder in an at-risk sample of high school adolescents: A randomized trial of a group cognitive intervention. *Journal of the American Academy of Child and Adolescent Psychiatry*, **34**, 312–321.

Clarke, G.N., Hornbrook, M., Lynch, F., Polen, M., Gale, J., Beardslee, W., *et al.* (2001). A randomized trial of a group cognitive intervention for preventing depression in adolescent offspring of depressed parents. *Archives of General Psychiatry*, **58**, 1127–1134.

Cohen, P., Pine, D.S., Must, A., Kasen, S., and Brook, J. (1998). Prospective associations between somatic illness and mental illness from childhood to adulthood. *American Journal of Epidemiology*, 147, 232–239.

Costello, E.J., Pine, D.S., Hammen, C., *et al.* (2001). Development and natural history of mood disorders. Unpublished manuscript.

Coyne, J.C., Burchill, S.A.L., and Stiles, W.B. (1991). An interactional perspective on depression. In C.R. Snyder and D.R. Forsyth (Eds.), *Handbook of Social and Clinical Psychology: The Health Perspective*. Pergamon Press, New York, pp. 327–349.

Farmer, R., and Nelson-Gray, R.O. (1990). Personality disorders and depression: Hypothetical relations, empirical findings, and methodological considerations. *Clinical Psychology Review*, 10, 453–475.

Fava, M., Abraham, M., Alpert, J., Nierenberg, A.A., Pava, J.A., and Rosenbaum, J.F. (1996). Gender differences in Axis 1 comorbidity among depressed outpatients. *Journal of Affective Disorders*, 38, 129–133.

Fleming, J.E. and Offord, D.R. (1990). Epidemiology of childhood depressive disorders: A critical review. *Journal of the American Academy of Child and Adolescent Psychiatry*, 29, 571–580.

Garber, J., Kriss, M.R., Koch, M., and Lindholm, L. (1988). Recurrent depression in adolescents: A follow-up study. *Journal of the American Academy of Child and Adolescent Psychiatry*, 27, 49–54.

Geller, B., Zimerman, B., Williams, M., Bolhofner, K., and Craney, J.L. (2001). Adult psychosocial outcome of prepubertal major depressive disorder. *Journal of the American Academy of Child and Adolescent Psychiatry*, 40, 673–677.

Gonzales, L.R., Lewinsohn, P.M., and Clarke, G.N. (1985). Longitudinal follow-up of unipolar depressives: An investigation of predictors of relapse. *Journal of Consulting and Clinical Psychology*, 53, 461–469.

Goodman, S.H., Lahey, B.B., Fielding, B., Dulcan, M., Narrow, W., and Regier, D. (1997). Representativeness of clinical samples of youths with mental disorders: A preliminary population-based study. *Journal of Abnormal Psychology*, 106, 3–14.

Goodyer, I.M., Herbert, J., Secher, S.M., and Pearson, J. (1997). Short-term outcome of major depression: I. Comorbidity and severity at presentation as predictors of persistent disorder. *Journal of the American Academy of Child and Adolescent Psychiatry*, 36, 179–187.

Gotlib, I.H., Lewinsohn, P.M., and Seeley, J.R. (1998). Consequences of depression during adolescence: Marital status and marital functioning in early adulthood. *Journal of Abnormal Psychology*, 107, 686–690.

Hammen, C. (1991). Generation of stress in the course of unipolar depression. *Journal of Abnormal Psychology*, 100, 555–561.

Hammen, C. (1999). The emergence of an interpersonal approach to depression. In T.E. Joiner, Jr. and J. Coyne (Eds.), *The Interactional Nature of Depression: Advances in Interpersonal Approaches*. American Psychological Association, Washington, DC, pp. 21–35.

Hammen, C. and Garber, J. (2001). Vulnerability to depression across the lifespan. In R.E. Ingram and J.M. Price (Eds.), *Vulnerability to Psychopathology: Risk Across the Lifespan*. Guilford, New York, pp. 258–267.

Harrington, R., Fudge, H., Rutter, M., Pickels, A., and Hill, J. (1990). Adult outcomes of childhood and adolescent depression: I. Psychiatric status. *Archives of General Psychiatry*, **47**, 465–473.

Harrington, R., Fudge, H., Rutter, M., Pickles, A., and Hill, J. (1991). Adult outcomes of childhood and adolescent depression: II. Links with antisocial disorders. *Journal of the American Academy of Child and Adolescent Psychiatry*, **30**, 434–439.

Hirschfeld, R.M.A., Klerman, G.L., Chodoff, P., Korchin, S., and Barrett, J. (1976). Dependency–self-esteem–clinical depression. *Journal of the American Academy of Psychoanalysis*, **4**, 373–388.

Hirschfeld, R.M.A., Klerman, G.L., Gough, H.G., Barrett, J., Korchin, S.J., and Chodoff, P. (1977). A measure of interpersonal dependency. *Journal of Personality Assessment*, **41**, 610–619.

Hirschfeld, R.M.A., Klerman, G.L., Lavori, P., Keller, M.B., Griffith, P., and Coryell, W. (1989). Premorbid personality assessments of first onset of major depression. *Archives of General Psychiatry*, **46**, 345–350.

Ilardi, S.S., Craighead, W.E., and Evans, D.D. (1997). Modeling relapse in unipolar depression: The effects of dysfunctional cognitions and personality disorders. *Journal of Consulting and Clinical Psychology*, **65**, 381–391.

Jaycox, L.H., Reivich, K.J., Gillham, J., and Seligman, M.E.P. (1994). Prevention of depressive symptoms in school children. *Behavior Research Therapy*, **32**, 801–816.

Kandel, D.B. and Davies, M. (1986). Adult sequella of adolescent depressive symptoms. *Archives of General Psychiatry*, **43**, 255–262.

Kashani, J.H., Carlson, G.A., Beck, N.C., *et al.* (1987). Depression, depressive symptoms, and depressed mood among a community sample of adolescents. *American Journal of Psychiatry*, **144**, 931–934.

Keller, M.B., Lavori, P.W., Beardslee, W.R., Wunder, J., and Ryan, N. (1991). Depression in children and adolescents: New data on 'undertreatment' and a literature review on the efficiency of available treatments. *Journal of Affective Disorders*, **21**, 163–171.

Keller, M.B., Lavori, P.W., Friedman, B., Nielsen, E., Endicott, J., and McDonald-Scott, P.A. (1987). The Longitudinal Interval Follow-up Evaluation: A comprehensive method for assessing outcome in prospective longitudinal studies. *Archives of General Psychiatry*, **44**, 540–548.

Kessler, R.C. (1997). The prevalence of psychiatric comorbidity. In S. Wetzler and W.C. Sanderson (Eds.), *Treatment Strategies for Patients with Psychiatric Comorbidity*. Wiley, New York, pp. 23–48.

Kessler, R.C., Berglund, P.A., Foster, C.L., Saunders, W.B., Stang, P.E., and Walters, E.E. (1997). The social consequences of psychiatric disorders: II. Teenage parenthood. *American Journal of Psychiatry*, **154**, 1405–1411.

Kessler, R.C. and Frank, R.G. (1996). The impact of psychiatric disorders on work loss days. *Psychological Medicine*, **27**, 861–873.

Kessler, R.C., McGonagle, K.A., Swartz, M., Blazer, D.G., and Nelson, C.B. (1993). Sex and depression in the National Comorbidity Survey I: Lifetime prevalence, chronicity, and recurrence. *Journal of Affective Disorders*, **29**, 85–96.

Kessler, R.C., Walters, E.E., and Forthofer, M.S. (1998). The social consequences of psychiatric disorders, III: Probability of marital stability. *American Journal of Psychiatry*, **155**, 1092–1096.

Kovacs, M., Feinberg, T.L., Crouse-Novack, M.A., Paulauskas, S.L., and Finkelstein, R. (1984). Depressive disorders in childhood I: A longitudinal prospective study of characteristics and recovery. *Archives of General Psychiatry*, **41**, 229–237.

Kovacs, M., Feinberg, T.L., Crouse-Novack, M.A., Paulauskas, S.L., Pollock, M., and Finkelstein, R. (1984). Depressive disorders in childhood. II: A longitudinal study of the risk for a subsequent major depression. *Archives of General Psychiatry*, **41**, 643–649.

Lewinsohn, P.M., Allen, N.B., Seeley, J.R., and Gotlib, I.H. (1999*a*). First onset versus recurrence of depression: Differential processes of psychosocial risk. *Journal of Abnormal Psychology*, **108**, 483–489.

Lewinsohn, P.M., Hops, H., Roberts, R.E., Seeley, J.R., and Andrews, J.A. (1993). Adolescent psychopathology: I. Prevalence and incidence of depression and other DSM-III-R disorders in high school students. *Journal of Abnormal Psychology*, **102**, 133–144.

Lewinsohn, P.M., Pettit, J., Joiner, T.E., Jr, and Seeley, J.R. (2001*a*). Phenomenology of adolescent depression. Unpublished manuscript.

Lewinsohn, P.M., Roberts, R.E., Seeley, J.R., Rohde, P., Gotlib, I.H., and Hops, H. (1994). Adolescent psychopathology: II. Psychosocial risk factors for depression. *Journal of Abnormal Psychology*, **103**, 302–315.

Lewinsohn, P.M., Rohde, P., Klein, D.N., and Seeley, J.R. (1999*b*). Natural course of adolescent major depressive disorder: I. Continuity into young adulthood. *Journal of the American Academy of Child and Adolescent Psychiatry*, **38**, 56–63.

Lewinsohn, P.M., Rohde, P., and Seeley, J.R. (1998). Treatment of adolescent depression: Frequency of services and impact on functioning in young adulthood. *Depression and Anxiety*, **7**, 47–52.

Lewinsohn, P.M., Rohde, P., Seeley, J.R., and Baldwin, C.L. (2001*b*). Gender differences in suicide attempts from adolescence to young adulthood. *Journal of the American Academy of Child and Adolescent Psychiatry*, **40**, 427–434.

Lewinsohn, P.M., Rohde, P., Seeley, J.R., Klein, D.N., and Gotlib, I. (2001*c*). Psychosocial impairment of young adults who have experienced and recovered from major depressive disorder during adolescence. Unpublished manuscript.

Lewinsohn, P.M., Rohde, P., Seeley, J.R., Klein, D.N., and Gotlib, I.H. (2000). Natural course of adolescent major depressive disorder in a community sample: Predictors of recurrence in young adults. *American Journal of Psychiatry*, **157**, 1584–1591.

Lewinsohn, P.M., Sullivan, J.M., and Grosscup, S.J. (1982). Behavioral therapy: Clinical applications. In A.J. Rush (Ed.), *Short-term Psychotherapies for the Depressed Patient*. Guilford Press, New York, pp. 50–87.

Mannuzza, S. and Fyer, A.J. (1990). *Family informant schedule and criteria (FISC), July 1990 revision*. New York, Anxiety Disorders Clinic, New York State Psychiatric Institute.

McGee, R., Feehan, M., Williams, S., Partridge, F., Silva, P.A., and Kelly, J. (1990). DSM-III disorders in a large sample of adolescents. *Journal of the American Academy of Child and Adolescent Psychiatry*, **29**, 611–619.

Merikangas, K.R., Wicki, W., and Angst, J. (1994). Heterogeneity of depression: Classification of depressive subtypes by longitudinal course. *British Journal of Psychiatry*, **164**, 342–348.

Miranda, J. and Persons, J.B. (1988). Dysfunctional attitudes are mood-state dependent. *Journal of Abnormal Psychology*, **97**, 76–79.

Miranda, J., Persons, J.B., and Byers, C.N. (1990). Endorsement of dysfunctional beliefs depends on current mood state. *Journal of Abnormal Psychology*, **99**, 237–241.

Monroe, S.M., Rohde, P., Seeley, J.R., and Lewinsohn, P.M. (1999). Life events and depression in adolescence: Relationship loss as a prospective risk factor for first onset of major depressive disorder. *Journal of Abnormal Psychology*, **108**, 606–614.

Mrazek, P.J. and Haggerty, R.J. (1994). *Reducing Risks for Mental Disorders: Frontiers for Preventive Intervention Research*. National Academy Press, Washington, DC.

Offord, D.R., Boyle, M.H., Szatmari, P., *et al.* (1987). Ontario Child Health Study: II. Six month prevalence of disorder and rates of service utilization. *Archives of General Psychiatry*, **44**, 832–836.

Oldham, J.M., Skodol, A.E., Kellman, H.D., Hyler, S.E., Doidge, N., Rosnick, L., and Gallagher, P.E. (1995). Comorbidity of Axis I and Axis II disorders. *American Journal of Psychiatry*, **152**, 571–578.

Orvaschel, H., Puig-Antich, J., Chambers, W.J., Tabrizi, M.A., and Johnson, R. (1982). Retrospective assessment of prepubertal major depression with the Kiddie-SADS-E. *Journal of the American Academy of Child Psychiatry*, **21**, 392–397.

Pine, D.S., Cohen, P., Ma, Y., Gurley, D., Brook, J., and Ma, Y. (1998). The risk for early-adulthood anxiety and depressive disorders in adolescents with anxiety and depressive disorders. *Archives of General Psychiatry*, **55**, 56–64.

Post, R.M. (1992). Transduction of psychosocial stress into the neurobiology of recurrent affective disorder. *American Journal of Psychiatry*, **149**, 999–1010.

Post, R.M., Weiss, S.B., and Leverich, G.S. (1994). Recurrent affective disorder: Roots in developmental neurobiology and illness progression based on changes in gene expression. *Development and Psychopathology*, **6**, 781–813.

Post, R.M., Weiss, S.R.B., Leverich, G.S., George, M.S., Frye, M., and Ketter, T.A. (1996). Developmental psychobiology of cyclic affective illness: Implications for early therapeutic intervention. *Development and Psychopathology*, **8**, 273–305.

Rao, U., Hammen, C., and Daley, S.E. (1999). Continuity of depression during the transition to adulthood: A 5-year longitudinal study of young women. *Journal of the American Academy of Child and Adolescent Psychiatry*, **38**, 908–915.

Rao, U., Ryan, N.D., Birmaher, B., *et al.* (1995). Unipolar depression in adolescents: Clinical outcomes in adulthood. *Journal of the American Academy of Child Psychiatry*, **34**, 566–578.

Reinherz, H., Giaconia, R.M., Carmola, A.M., Wasserman, M.W., and Silverman, A.B. (1999b). Major depression in young adulthood: Risks and impairments. *Journal of Abnormal Psychology*, **108**, 500–510.

Reinherz, H.Z., Giaconia, R.M., Hauf, A.M.C., Wasserman, M.S., and Silverman, A.B. (1999a). Major depression in the transition to adulthood: Risks and impairments. *Journal of Abnormal Psychology*, **108**, 500–510.

Rohde, P., Lewinsohn, P.M., and Seeley, J.R. (1991). Comorbidity of unipolar depression: II Comorbidity with other mental disorders in adolescents and adults. *Journal of Abnormal Psychology*, **100**, 214–222.

Rohde, P., Lewinsohn, P.M., and Seeley, J.R. (1994). Are adolescents changed by an episode of major depression? *Journal of the American Academy of Child and Adolescent Psychiatry*, **33**, 1289–1298.

Skodol, A.E., Stout, R.L., McGlashan, T.H., *et al.* (1999). The co-occurrence of mood and personality disorders: A report from the Collaborative Longitudinal Personality Disorders Study (CLPS). *Depression and Anxiety*, **10**, 175–182.

Teasdale, J.D. (1983). Negative thinking in depression: Cause, effect or reciprocal relationship? *Advances in Behavior Research and Therapy*, **5**, 3–25.

Teasdale, J.D. (1988). Cognitive vulnerability to persistent depression. *Cognition and Emotion*, **2**, 247–274.

Teasdale, J.D. and Dent, J. (1987). Cognitive vulnerability to depression: An investigation of two hypotheses. *British Journal of Clinical Psychology*, **26**, 113–126.

Velez, C.N., Johnson, J., and Cohen, P. (1989). A longitudinal analysis of selected risk factors for childhood psychopathology. *Journal of the American Academy of Child and Adolescent Psychiatry*, **28**, 861–864.

Verhulst, F.C., Van Der Ende, J., Ferdinand, R.F., and Kasius, M.C. (1997). The prevalence of DSM-III-R diagnoses in a national sample of Dutch adolescents. *Archives of General Psychiatry*, **54**, 329–336.

Warner, V., Weissman, M.M., Fendrich, M., Wickramaratne, P., and Moreau, D. (1992). The course of major depression in the offspring of depressed parents: Incidence, recurrence, and recovery. *Archives of General Psychiatry*, **49**, 795–801.

Weissman, M.M. and Paykel, E.S. (1974). *The Depressed Woman*. University of Chicago Press, Chicago.

Weissman, M.M., Wolk, S., Goldstein, R.B., *et al.* (1999). Depressed adolescents grown up. *Journal of the American Medical Association*, **281**, 1707–1713.

Winokur, G. and Tsuang, M.T. (1996). *The Natural History of Mania, Depression, and Schizophrenia*. American Psychiatric Press, Washington, DC.

Youngren, M. and Lewinsohn, P.M. (1980). The functional relation between depression and problematic interpersonal behavior. *Journal of Abnormal Psychology*, **89**, 333–341.

Chapter 6

Depression in midlife

E. S. Paykel and N. Kennedy

This chapter is concerned with depression between the ages of forty and
sixty. The median age of most adult samples of depressed patients is in the
forties. This is the core age for depression research, involving the largest
number of studies, and forms the anchor group to which other age groups
are compared. Surprisingly little has been written about specific features
of depression in middle age, or about midlife problems. We will highlight
aspects which are relevant to the life cycle or are currently timely and we
will make some comparisons with other adult age groups.

Epidemiology

Depression is common in the community and not all cases present to doc-
tors. Reliable data on the prevalence became established with application
of standardized criteria and case finding instruments in community surveys in the 1980s and 1990s. Six-month prevalence rates for major depression are in the range 2–6 per cent (Smith and Weissman, 1992). There are
variations between different centres and countries but it is unclear how
much these depend on methodological factors, cultural interview response
styles, differences in the terms used for emotions in translated interviews
in different languages, or substantive factors.

Lifetime incidence for major depression is less well established, with figures varying widely from 2 to 20 per cent or more, higher in women than
men. Figures for dysthymia are probably more reliable due to its persistence,
and are of the order of 2–4 per cent. Lifetime figures for bipolar disorder
are also probably more reliable, due to its greater severity, recurrence and
likelihood of treatment, and are around 1 per cent.

The US National Comorbidity Survey focussed on co-occurrence of
other disorders. Eleven per cent of those with a lifetime episode of major

depression also had an episode of panic disorder; 56 per cent of those with panic disorder had major depression (Roy-Byrne *et al.*, 2000). Often these occurred together.

There has been a debate as to whether lifetime incidence of depression is rising. A number of studies have reported increased rates. However these mainly depend on retrospective reporting in cross-sectional surveys, a method which may not be reliable (Andrews *et al.*, 1999). In these studies comparisons are made between age-stratified rates in younger subjects and those reported retrospectively by the elderly. If the elderly forget the depression of their youth or never interpreted it as depression, rates may be spuriously low (Paykel, 2000). More reliable data are obtained from systematic lifetime studies of more than one cohort. The Lundby study (Hagnell *et al.*, 1982) has found increased rates in younger males, while the Stirling County study has not found clear increase (Murphy *et al.*, 2000).

With respect to age, prevalence, and incidence of major depression extend across adulthood (Smith and Weissman, 1992). First onset of bipolar disorder tends to be younger, as does dysthymia. Community studies from Canberra suggest some decline in community prevalence in old age, but also suggest that symptoms may change (Jorm, 2000).

Unipolar depression consistently shows a female preponderance of 2 : 1 or greater, both in treated and in community samples, while sex ratios are more equal in bipolar disorder. There is some evidence that the sex ratio for unipolar disorder is highest in middle age (Jorm, 1987). Reasons for the female preponderance are not clear but probably include both biological and social factors (Paykel, 1991). Biological mechanisms, such as hormonal effects on the brain, although plausible are hard to investigate. Epidemiological studies indicate that much of the excess occurs in married women aged 25–54 years with children, strongly suggesting social causes related to the vulnerable situation of young mothers. Some studies suggest the effect is primarily due to children (Gater *et al.*, 1989). The significance of marriage itself has changed in an era of less formal cohabitation and single motherhood. Differential gender acknowledgement and direction of distress may play a part. Any differences in help-seeking play only a minor role.

Although rates of major depression are higher in married women in younger adulthood, later, and in males, they are highest in the single, widowed, divorced, and bereaved. They tend to be higher in more deprived socioeconomic groups in community samples, less so in treated samples and in bipolar disorder. There is a trend to higher rates in urban residents (Paykel *et al.*, 2000) but not in all studies.

Clinical features

Most of those who present for the first time with clinical depression do so in early or middle adult life. As a consequence diagnostic and classification systems have been based on this group. The clinical features of depression are dealt with well in standard textbooks and do not need recapitulation here. The two standard classifications, the International Classification of Disorders (ICD-10) and the American Psychiatric Association Diagnostic and Statistical Manual (DSM-IV) have converged somewhat in their most recent editions, although there are still considerable differences of detail. Both highlight the bipolar–unipolar distinction, which is now regarded as the most clear-cut and important one within affective disorders. Both assign a subclassification for psychotic depression (presence of delusions or hallucinations). This is particularly valuable for treatment, since it often does not respond well to antidepressants alone, and better to ECT or to antidepressant–neuroleptic combinations. Both also retain what formerly was called 'endogenous' depression, as a symptom picture, labelled somatic syndrome in ICD-10, melancholia in DSM-IV. A major difference is in organization, with ICD-10 using a division into single episode, recurrent disorder, and persistent disorders, while DSM-IV assigns primacy to the bipolar–unipolar distinction. Classification depending on single vs recurrent disorder has problems, since many of the former ultimately become the latter. Dysthymia has become well established since its introduction to nosology 20 years ago, and defines a well recognized long term disorder, often punctuated by superimposed major depressive episodes.

Differences have been reported in clinical symptoms, with elderly subjects having less depressed mood than midlife depressives but more anxiety (Gottfries, 1998) and more somatic complaints, whether due to somatization or accentuation of comorbid physical illness. Cognitive dysfunction is often seen in depression in the elderly and can be difficult to distinguish from true dementia. Biological symptoms, suspiciousness, ideas of reference, and persecutory or hypochondriacal beliefs occur more frequently in the elderly (Brodaty et al., 1997). Negative cognitive beliefs, such as feelings of guilt and pessimism, as well as loss of interest and sleep difficulties, have also been reported as being more frequent in elderly subjects (Koenig et al., 1993).

Some other studies have shown few or minor differences in symptoms between older and younger depressives (Hermann et al., 1989). A recent study comparing symptomatology in 461 younger and elderly inpatients found significantly more agitation and hypochondriasis in elderly inpatients, but the differences were small (Stage et al., 2001).

An episode of depression in midlife may represent a first episode or more commonly recurrence of an established depressive illness. Klein *et al.* (1999), studying outpatients with chronic major depression found that compared with depression starting in midlife, depression with an early onset was associated with a longer index episode, higher rates of recurrence and hospitalization, comorbid personality disorder, substance use disorder and depressive personality traits but no differences were found in clinical symptoms, symptom severity, functional impairment or treatment response. Comorbid psychiatric disorders and personality disorders have been associated more strongly with early onset, particularly onset during childhood or adolescence (Alpert *et al.*, 1999).

Childhood depression is discussed in Chapter 2. Compared with children, adolescents have more typical symptoms resembling those seen in adults (Ryan *et al.*, 1987).

Aetiology: life stress

Depression is multifactorial in origin in all age groups, with causative factors and mechanisms ranging through genes, other biological and neuro-endocrine mechanisms, early environment, recent life stress, and social support. All must be presumed to come together in a final common pathway in neural systems regulating mood.

Among these, life stress has been well studied. Systematic studies of recent life events have been undertaken since the late 1960s, and have been reviewed extensively (Paykel and Cooper, 1992; Paykel, 1994*a*, 2001*a*). Few studies are limited to middle-aged samples but these subjects predominate in sample characteristics.

A large number of comparisons with general population, psychiatric and other controls, show raised rates of stressful life events independent of the subject's causation in the six months or longer prior to the onset of depression, particularly in the most recent three months. The literature lays particular emphasis on loss events or interpersonal exits, but a wide range of other events which can be viewed as stressful, threatening, distressing or negative appear also to be involved.

There is also a large literature on social support (Brugha, 1995). Although study has been less rigorous than for life events, studies in depression show negative effects of absence of support and beneficial effects of its presence (Paykel and Cooper, 1992). It has been argued whether the effect is primarily due to buffering of stressful life events or is independent: probably it is both (Cohen and Wills, 1985). Social support may not be independent of the individual since personality may strongly influence the size and intimacy of personal social networks.

There has been little attempt in these studies to focus separately on the events of middle age. This is the portion of the life cycle where moves, job changes, and marital breakdowns are less frequent than before forty, but may be more catastrophic when they do occur. It is also a time when people need to come to terms with failed aspirations for careers or other life aspects, when children achieve adulthood and leave home, forcing readjustments on parents and on marriages. One's own parents become elderly and infirm, and this may throw heavy burden on carers, particularly middle-aged daughters. Physical changes of middle age occur. Males become aware of decline in physical fitness, of middle-aged spread. Women experience the menopause with its troublesome flushes for some, and its signal of the end of childbearing—which may as often be welcomed as it is regretted. Physical illness starts to become more common. Increasingly, by the fifties, retirement from work begins to occur, most often in this life period forced by job loss or illness. This may also be a time of increased financial commitment to pay for children's higher education.

There is an overall trend in studies of life events and depression for fewer events to occur as age increases. This also applies to control samples, and appears to reflect a general tendency for lives to become more stable in middle age. There is no clear-cut evidence as to how the magnitude of life stress effects on depression vary with age, but life stress has been found to precede old age depression in controlled studies (Emmerson et al., 1989). Where genetic effects are strong they are often thought to bring forward to an earlier age the onset of disorder. This has been found for bipolar disorder (Johnson et al., 2000) but there is not clear evidence for unipolar depression. Life events do tend to be more important in earlier episodes of depression than later (Johnson et al., 2000; Kendler et al., 2000). Magnitude of genetic loading and amount of life stress have been hypothesized to correlate inversely in depression, but evidence is not consistent (Paykel, 2001a).

In addition to its influence on the onset of adult depression life stress influences the course (Paykel and Cooper, 1992). Remission appears to be more common where positive events such as 'fresh start' events occur (Brown et al., 1988), and less common with negative events, and relapse or recurrence subsequently more common with negative events. The exception is where depression is both severe and already recurrent, where two studies have not found stress to influence outcome on follow-up (Andrew et al., 1993; Paykel et al., 1996).

There has been a longstanding debate, now less active, regarding the so-called endogenous depression. The concept involves not only presence or absence of life stress, but also a symptom pattern now most commonly referred to, from DSM-III and its successors, as melancholia. While some depressions, particularly recurrent ones, appear unrelated to life stress and others highly related to it, the relation between this and the melancholic symptom pattern, or to psychotic depression with depressive delusions, appears quite weak, although tending to be in the expected direction (Paykel and Cooper, 1992).

In recent years work has extended to the origins of life events (Paykel, 2001a) with findings which bear on a lifespan approach. Events are not merely accidental occurrences. Hammen (1991) studied dependent rather than events rated independent of illness, and as expected found them more common in unipolar depressives than normal controls. There were no differences for independent events. Harkness *et al.* (1999) found dependent events more common in recurrent depressives than in first episodes. These events, although generated partly by depression, may be important themselves in producing further episodes.

There is a growing strain of research examining familial and genetic elements in generation of events. McGuffin *et al.* (1988) found raised event rates in family members of depressives, although this could have been environmental in origin including shared social environment. Plomin *et al.* (1990) found higher correlations in monozygotic than dizygotic twins for life events over the whole lifespan. Farmer *et al.* (2001) in a sib pair design found only weak relationships between sensation seeking scores and life events, mainly due to non-severe events rather than the severe events associated with depression.

Kendler and colleagues have made productive use of the large Virginia twin registry to explore genetic and environmental elements. Using postal questionnaire reports of occurrence of forty-four life events in the past year, Kendler *et al.* (1993) found correlations which were a little higher in monozygotic twins than dizygotic. Genetic and environmental elements each accounted for about 20 per cent of the variance with the genetic element predominant in 'network' events affecting individuals in the respondent's social networks, and the environmental element in 'personal' events directly affecting the respondent. Later information was collected by interview. Genetic influences affected liability to develop depression after life events (Kendler *et al.*, 1995). Genetic liability to major depression increased the risk of being exposed to life events, mainly personal ones, outside the depressive episode (Kendler and Karkowski-Shuman, 1997). About one third of the relationship between life events and depression appeared to be non-causal, due to self-selection into high-risk environments (Kendler *et al.*, 1999a). No evidence was found for genetic effects on independent events of personal or network classes, but the latter showed considerable effects of familial environment (Kendler *et al.*, 1999b). Dependent events of both classes showed genetic effects.

Longitudinal studies have shown continuities from earlier life. In a very long term follow-up. Champion *et al.* (1995) found that children who had shown emotional or behavioural disturbance aged ten, when studied in their late twenties had markedly higher rates of highly threatening events and difficulties, both dependent and independent. Van Os and Jones (1999), using the British longitudinal 1946 birth cohort study, found that stressful life events in midlife were predicted by high neuroticism in childhood. This measure also predicted stronger effects of life events on disorder, which were also predicted by poorer childhood mental health and higher maternal neuroticism in the subjects' childhood.

Vaillant *et al.* (1998) found social support at ages 50–70 strongly predicted by alcohol abuse, smoking, and depression at age fifty. Long term longitudinal studies such as these three provide the best way of studying effects of early vulnerability factors.

Genetics

Much of the literature on the genetics of affective disorders deals with bipolar disorder and is not relevant to this volume. Genetic elements appear to be stronger in bipolar disorder than unipolar.

Evidence on unipolar depression from adoption studies has been equivocal to date (Sullivan *et al.*, 2000), with only one positive study supporting a genetic effect on the transmission of major depression. Twin studies of major depression show higher concordance rate for monozygotic twins suggesting a genetic influence (Kendler and Prescott, 1999). A meta-analysis of twin studies in major depression found 37 per cent of variance in liability for major depression due to genetic effects, 63 per cent due to individual-specific environmental (Sullivan *et al.*, 2000).

Transmission is likely to be multigenic, with combined effects from many genes. Recent years have seen a vigorous search for genes using linkage and candidate gene molecular genetic approaches. Replication of findings has been difficult and effect of individual genes in general appears weak. Linkage studies have mainly been concerned with bipolar disorder.

In candidate gene approaches, genes involved in regulation, metabolism, and production of serotonin, noradrenaline, dopamine or their precursors have been most widely studied. Findings that major depression and suicide are associated with reduced serotonin uptake function (Collier *et al.*, 1996) and fewer serotonin transporter sites (Mann *et al.*, 2000) have led to findings that serotonin transporter gene polymorphisms (HTTLPR) are associated with affective disorder (Collier *et al.*, 1996) particularly major depression (Ogilvie *et al.*, 1996; Mann *et al.*, 2000) and violent suicide attempts (Bellivier *et al.*, 2000). However some studies have been negative. Allelic variation in the serotonin transporter and transporter promoter regions have been associated with response to SSRIs (Pollock *et al.*, 2000). Suicidal behaviour has been related to polymorphisms of the tryptophan hydroxylase gene in several studies (Abbar *et al.*, 2001), again with negative studies. Similarly associations have been found between polymorphisms of monoamine oxidase genes and depression (Rubinsztein *et al.*, 1996; Qian *et al.*, 1999, Schulze *et al.*, 2000), but negative studies have also been reported. Other positive associations with unipolar depression recently reported include polymorphisms of the dopamine D3 receptor (Dikeos *et al.*, 1999) and D4 receptor (Manki *et al.*, 1996), in addition to a positive association between suicide attempts and an allele of tyrosine hydroxylase (Persson *et al.*, 1997). No association has been found between polymorphisms of a number of other candidate genes and depression, including the noradrenaline transporter and serotonin receptors. The candidate gene approach depends on careful case control matching and needs to be replicated in several populations before a firm association is established. In addition, multiple hypothesis testing may lead to positive associations by chance, with additional publication bias in favour of positive results.

Family aggregation of depression has been associated with early age of onset in a number of studies but with some negative studies (Sullivan *et al.*, 2000). Other associations of familial depression in some but not all studies include recurrent episodes, longer episode length, and greater impairment (Sullivan *et al.*, 2000).

Biological mechanisms

There is a large literature on neuroendocrine changes in depression, which reached its peak in the late 1980s. Challenge studies have shown blunting of growth hormone response to the alpha-2 adrenoceptor agonist clonidine (Checkley *et al.*, 1981). More consistent has been the finding of blunting of prolactin response to serotoninergic agonists such as tryptophan, clomipramine, and, less consistently, fenfluramine (Park *et al.*, 1996). Studies like these show changes in a neuroendocrine system, although it is less clear whether the findings are due to decreased receptor sensitivity or some other change in the system and whether they reflect causes, mechanisms, or secondary neuroendocrine consequences of depression.

An additional finding related to serotonin, is induction of depression by tryptophan depletion, through administration of a high amino acid drink lacking tryptophan. Lowered mood in recovering depressives, particularly those on serotoninergic antidepressants, and in some studies, in drug-free recovered depressives and normals with a positive family history of depression (Moore *et al.*, 2000; van der Does, 2001), strongly implicates a serotonin pathway in depression.

The most studied aspect has been the hypothalamic pituitary adrenal (HPA) axis, and the most consistent neuroendocrine abnormality in depression is hypersecretion of cortisol with impaired hypothalamic feedback. This has been found in studies of basal blood levels, 24-h blood levels, salivary levels, and studies of urinary excretion products. Earlier hopes that failure of dexamethasone suppression of cortisol would be specific were not sustained, since the abnormality is present in only 50 per cent of depressives even when showing melancholia, and also may be found to some extent in other psychoses, eating disorders and Alzheimer's disease. The DST non-suppression at remission does predict relapse (Ribeiro *et al.*, 1993). Some improvement in test characteristics can be obtained by combining dexamethasone with CRH stimulation (Heuser *et al.*, 1994). Age affects dexamethasone suppression, with higher post dexamethasone cortisol levels and greater likelihood of a positive test in older subjects (Davies *et al.*, 1984; Nelson *et al.*, 1984). Plasma levels of dexamethasone are also higher in older subjects (Hunt *et al.*, 1989).

Recently, an opposite hormonal abnormality of lowered dehydroepiandrosterone (DHEA) has been found in adult depressives (Michael *et al.*, 2000) confirming earlier findings in children. Salivary DHEA was lowered in major depressives at 8am and 8pm compared with normal controls, with remitted depressives intermediate, suggesting a state abnormality. Morning DHEA levels were inversely correlated with depression severity.

It has been suggested that HPA abnormalities may be involved in causative mechanisms. Animal studies have shown that early stress can alter the development of the HPA axis and other systems, and CRF has been proposed as a mediating factor for many of the changes (Kaufmann *et al.*, 2000). In young women who have been abused in childhood hyperresponsivity of the HPA axis to laboratory stressors has been found (Hein *et al.*, 2000). In depressives it has been suggested that HPA activity may contribute to depressed mood. There is some evidence that cortisol suppression with metyrapone, ketoconazole, aminoglutethimide or dexamethasone may improve depressed mood in clinical depressives (Murphy, 1997), although studies have been small scale and short term and effects do not appear to be large.

A growing area of biological research into neural substrates has been by neuroimaging, particularly functional neuroimaging by positron emission tomography (PET) and functional magnetic resonance imaging (fMRI). Structural imaging does not show consistent abnormalities in middle-aged depressives but there is emerging MRI evidence of reduction in subgenual prefrontal cortex (Drevets *et al.*, 1997) with histological glial reduction (Ongur *et al.*, 1998). There is also some evidence of left hippocampal reduction (Bremner *et al.*, 2000; Mervaala *et al.*, 2000). In elderly depressives there is increasing evidence of a group with white matter hyperintensities and impaired cognitive function, where aetiology may be vascular (see Chapter 7). Neuropsychological studies in adults, mainly middle-aged depressives, show deficits in executive function and response to negative feedback (Elliott *et al.*, 1996, 1997a). Functional imaging studies, particularly of blood flow by ^{15}O PET and fMRI combined with executive and other neuropsychological tasks, particularly point to reduced blood flow in anterior cingulate, caudate, limbic and frontal areas (Elliott *et al.*, 1997b, 1998).

Acute treatment with medication

Tricyclic antidepressants (TCAs), SSRIs, and the newer serotonin/noradrenaline reuptake inhibitors (SNRIs) appear to be equally efficacious in treating acute depression with choice on the basis of side effects and safety. However drugs that potentiate both serotonin and noradrenaline (e.g. amitriptyline, venlafaxine) may be more effective than SSRIs in patients with severe depressive symptoms (Anderson, 1997). In atypical depression, with reactive mood and reversed biological features, MAOIs may be superior to TCAs (Quitkin *et al.*, 1993). SSRIs have been found as effective as MAOIs in atypical depression (Pande *et al.*, 1996).

Some patients will have low plasma levels on 150 mg of a standard TCA and higher doses have been shown to be more effective in some patients (Simpson *et al.*, 1976). High doses around 250–300 mg/day are sometimes used, particularly in refractory depression, and more in the United States than Europe (Phillips and Nierenberg, 1994). Secondary amines (e.g. nortriptyline) give a curvilinear dose response curve, with a therapeutic window within which optimal response occurs, which may require measurement of plasma levels. Higher doses of MAOIs also produce better response and often very high dosage is required (Young *et al.*, 1986). Better response to venlafaxine is also seen at high dose (Kienke and Rosenbaum, 2000). Although SSRIs may show flatter dose response curves (Cowen, 1998), higher dosage may also produce better response in some patients.

The variety of antidepressants now available has led to greater differences between individual psychiatrists and between countries in drug choice. In most countries currently the first choice for mild to moderate depression is an SSRI. For more severe or non-responding depression choice varies with broader spectrum uptake inhibiting drugs more prominent.

Six weeks treatment has often been viewed as an adequate trial before considering a change of antidepressant but may be too short (Greenhouse *et al.*, 1987). Ideally, in depression in mid-life the aim should be to treat with high dose antidepressant for eight to twelve weeks before changing drugs, although in practice this can be difficult to achieve.

Thirty to forty per cent of patients will fail to respond to an adequate trial of an antidepressant, and an additional problem is partial response (Paykel *et al.*, 1995). After inadequate response, switching to an alternative antidepressant class is usually considered. Venlafaxine at high doses has been reported to show some superiority over SSRIs, particularly regarding full remission of symptoms (Methonen *et al.*, 2000) and also appears useful in refractory major depression (Poirier and Boyer, 1999)

Treatment resistant depression tends to be more common in mid and later life. Such patients are common in specialist psychiatric care. Patients with resistant depression require full assessment, with review of history, diagnosis adequacy of previous treatment, family and social setting, perpetuating social and personality factors, and medical illnesses. Hypothyroidism including subtle subclinical grades can contribute (Targum *et al.*, 1984) and may be a consequence of treatment with lithium. The presence of a comorbid personality disorder is associated with reduced response rates to antidepressant therapy (Pfohl *et al.*, 1984).

Treatment choices with medication involve changing to an alternative antidepressant and augmentation. Lithium augmentation of all major classes of antidepressants is best established with a cumulative response rate in ten placebo controlled trials in refractory patients of 48 per cent (Price *et al.*, 2001). Another augmentation strategy commonly utilized, but with less controlled trial evidence is addition of thyroxine or triiodothyronine. Triiodothyronine appears to be more effective (Thase and Rush, 1995). Pindolol and buspirone have also been used as augmentation agents, but without convincing results. Pindolol appears to accelerate response to SSRIs, but studies in resistant depression have been disappointing. Positive results from buspirone augmentation of antidepressants have been claimed in small open studies but recent controlled trials have failed to show significant benefit.

Neuroleptics have long been used in combination with antidepressants in treating psychotic or near-psychotic depression. Atypical neuroleptics have been investigated as augmentation agents in non-psychotic depression but studies are still preliminary.

Antidepressant combinations are widely used in resistant depression. Several small studies have reported response to combinations of SSRI and TCA, but SSRIs may also inhibit metabolism of TCAs leading to toxic adverse effects. Combinations of MAOI and TCA are still occasionally used, with caution, and avoidance of serotoninergic TCAs such as clomipramine, and of SSRIs, so as not to produce a serotonin syndrome.

Finally electroconvulsive therapy (ECT) remains an important treatment choice in severe, psychotic or resistant depression. Benefits are greatest where depressive delusions and psychomotor retardation are present (Brandon *et al.*, 1984)

Continuation and maintenance treatment

It has become customary to distinguish two phases in treatment with medication beyond the acute episode: continuation treatment for six to nine months after remission and maintenance, for longer periods after this phase. In parallel, early symptom return has been termed relapse and distinguished from later occurrence of a new episode, or recurrence (Frank *et al.*, 1991). Numerous placebo controlled trials in depression demonstrate high rates of early relapse if antidepressants are withdrawn early after three months, markedly reduced by continuation for longer periods (Paykel, 2001*b*). This is routine practice in treatment of adult depression. Older recommendations were for at least four months after remission which should be complete because of high relapse rates in those with residual symptoms (Paykel *et al.*, 1995). There is evidence from a staged withdrawal controlled trial that this may be too short (Reimherr *et al.*, 1998) and clinical practice is now tending to longer periods of around nine months, with gradual withdrawal over two to three months to avoid withdrawal symptoms (Schatzberg *et al.*, 1997) or the possibility of rebound relapse.

Maintenance treatment is not routine but is indicated in depressives with several recurrences, particularly if these have been recent or there is other evidence of high risk. There is evidence of efficacy both of antidepressants and of lithium in preventing recurrence in unipolar depression (Paykel, 2001*b*). The most common maintenance treatment in practice is continuance of the antidepressant which led to recovery. Appropriate length of maintenance is less well established from controlled trials. In recurrent depressives recurrence rates may be high even after three years' maintenance following the continuation phase. Repeated recurrence on withdrawal is an indication for indefinite maintenance.

Age has not been critically examined in continuation and maintenance studies but there is evidence of benefit in the elderly (Georgotas *et al.*, 1989; Old Age Depression Interest Group, 1993; Reynolds *et al.*, 1999).

Psychological treatments

The place of psychological treatments in middle aged depression has become increasingly well established by good quality controlled trials.

There have been a small number of studies of group therapy, marital therapy, family therapy, and social work, indicating benefit in acute depression, but the largest number of studies has been of interpersonal therapy (IPT) and cognitive therapy (CBT). These are reviewed in detail elsewhere (Paykel, 1994*b*, 2001*b*).

Controlled trials of IPT in acute treatment show clear benefit (Paykel, 1994*b*). However in longer term use one trial showed no effect in preventing relapse after antidepressant withdrawal, but benefit on interpersonal relationships and social adjustment, a target of the psychotherapy (Paykel *et al.*, 1976). One study of acute and maintenance IPT in recurrence prevention showed only a weak effect, compared with strong effects from not withdrawing imipramine (Frank *et al.*, 1990), but another study has shown moderate benefit in elderly subjects, additive with nortriptyline (Reynolds *et al.*, 1999).

There is a rapidly growing literature on CBT, indicating benefit in acute depression, particularly in the milder range (Paykel, 1994*b*). One study found it suggestively inferior to IPT (Elkin *et al.*, 1992). A recent development has been several controlled trials showing prevention of relapse and recurrence, particularly where residual symptoms are present (Fava *et al.*, 1994; Paykel *et al.*, 1999; Teasdale *et al.*, 2000; Jarrett *et al.*, 2001). Prevention of further episodes appears to be emerging as a particularly beneficial effect of CBT.

Most studies of psychological therapies in acute treatment have been carried out in mildly or moderately depressed subjects, in the outpatient range or in general practice, and there is little evidence of clear benefit in severe or inpatient depressives, for whom there is good evidence of benefit from antidepressants and ECT. The evidence as to whether combinations of medication and psychological treatments produce additional benefit over one treatment alone is not consistent and effects may vary with the circumstances, the treatment, and the outcome measure. There is some evidence that benefit from combinations occurs with IPT (Paykel, 1994*b*; DiMascio *et al.*, 1979; Reynolds *et al.*, 1999) and with CBT in preventing relapse and residual depression (Paykel *et al.*, 1999). There is no evidence of deleterious effect from combination.

Psychological treatments have often been thought of in the past as particularly benefiting younger patients, but in fact benefits appear to extend fully across the adult age range. There is good evidence of benefit in the elderly from IPT in preventing recurrence and from CBT in acute treatment.

Natural history, course and outcome

In its delineation by Kraepelin affective disorder was regarded as a recurrent disorder. Many follow-ups in the first four decades of the twentieth century showed high recurrence rates (Robins and Guze, 1972). By the early 1960s, with the advent of modern treatments, good outcome tended to be assumed, but few follow-up studies were published. More recently the pendulum has swung back and high rates of recurrence have been emphasized.

Key findings were published in the 1980s. Early follow-up data from the NIMH Psychobiology Study (Keller *et al.*, 1984) showed moderately higher remission rates but a relapse rate of 35 per cent the year following remission. Later expansion of the study (Mueller *et al.*, 1999) found that over fifteen years 85 per cent of recovered subjects experienced a recurrence although only 58 per cent of those who remained well for five years did so. Two 16-year follow-up studies of inpatients (Kiloh *et al.*, 1988; Lee and Murray, 1988) showed that two-thirds had been readmitted, with an additional proportion having recurrences not requiring readmission. A review of earlier follow-up studies showed about 15 per cent of deaths due to suicide (Robins and Guze, 1972). Mortality is also raised due to cardiac and other deaths (Harris and Barraclough, 1998).

More recent studies have confirmed these trends. Remission rates on acute treatment are good, with only a comparatively small proportion showing resistant depression or chronicity (Ramana *et al.*, 1995). Relapse and recurrence rates are high (Paykel, 2001*b*). Suicide rates in follow-up studies appear to have fallen in samples treated since the 1940s (O'Leary *et al.*, 2001), which may indicate benefits from use of ECT, antidepressants and lithium.

Less adequate treatment following the acute episode has been found associated with higher relapse rates in some US studies (Dawson *et al.*, 1998) but the one British study (Ramana *et al.*, 1999) found relatively small deficiencies in continuing treatment which did not explain the high rates of episode return.

The influence of advancing age on outcome is reviewed in Chapter 7. Depression in the elderly has generally been considered to have worse prognosis than depression in midlife (Alexopoulos *et al.*, 1996) with high rates of suicide (Koenig and Blazer, 1992), in addition to raised mortality from other causes (Cole *et al.*, 1999). Subcortical white matter lesions on MRI have been found associated with poor prognosis (O'Brien *et al.*, 1998) and may be linked to dementia (Greenwald *et al.*, 1997). Poor prognosis in the elderly compared to midlife, may also be due to negative life events such as bereavement in addition to declining social supports and declining physical health (Koenig and Blazer, 1992). In addition elderly depressives are less likely to have their depression adequately recognized or to seek or receive adequate treatment (Coryell *et al.*, 1995).

However some studies, particularly treatment studies, show similar outcome in middle aged and older subjects. Remission rates, relapse rates and full recovery rates have been found similar in 'young old' patients (mean age sixty-eight years) and middle aged patients, treated with combined medication and psychological treatment (Reynolds *et al.*, 1996).

Considering prognostic factors worse outcome with slower remission is consistently predicted by more severe and longer illness and further episodes by previous recurrences (Ramana *et al.*, 1995). Residual symptoms are the strongest predictor of relapse (Paykel *et al.*, 1995). Few individual symptoms predict outcome. However negative self-esteem and abnormal personality profiles have been associated with poor short term outcome (Andrew *et al.*, 1993). Psychotic depression has a poorer outcome than non-psychotic depression with increased severity of episodes, longer episodes, greater incapacity and more relapses, and recurrences (Lee and Murray, 1988; Coryell *et al.*, 1996). Presence of thought disorder in psychotic depression has been associated with early relapse (Wilcox *et al.*, 2000).

References

Abbar, M., Courtet, P., Bellivier, F., *et al.* (2001). Suicide attempts and the tryptophan hydroxylase gene. *Molecular Psychiatry*, **6**, 268–273.

Alexopoulos, G.S., Meyers, B.S., Young, R.C., *et al.* (1996). Recovery in geriatric depression. *Archives of General Psychiatry*, **53**, 305–312.

Alpert, J.E., Fava, M., Uebelacker, L.A., *et al.* (1999). Patterns of axis 1 comorbidity in early-onset versus late-onset major depressive disorder. *Biological Psychiatry*, **46**, 202–211.

Anderson, I. (1997). Lessons to be learnt from meta-analysis of newer versus older antidepressants. *Advances in Psychiatric Treatment*, **3**, 58–63.

Andrew, B., Hawton, K., Fagg, J., and Westbrook, D. (1993). Do psychosocial factors influence outcome in severely depressed female psychiatric in-patients? *British Journal of Psychiatry*, **163**, 747–754.

Andrews, G., Anstey, K., Brodaty, H., Issakidis, C., and Luscombe, G. (1999). Recall of depressive episode 25 years previously. *Psychological Medicine*, **29**, 787–791.

Bellivier, F., Szoke, A., Henry, C., *et al.* (2000). Possible association between serotonin trannsporter gene polymorphism and violent suicidal behavior in mood disorders. *Biological Psychiatry*, **48**, 319–322.

Brandon, S., Cowley, P., McDonald, C., Neville, P., Palmer, R., and Wellstood-Eason, S. (1984). Electroconvulsive therapy: results in depressive illness from the Leicestershire trial. *British Medical Journal*, **288**, 22–25.

Bremner, J.D., Narayan, M., Anderson, E.R., Staib, L.H., Miller, H.L., and Charney, D.S. (2000). Hippocampal volume reduction in major depression. *American Journal of Psychiatry*, **157**, 115–117.

Brodaty, H., Luscombe, G., Parker, G., Wilhelm, K., Hickie, I., Austin, M.-P., and Mitchell, P. (1997). Increased rate of psychosis and psychomotor change in depression with age. *Psychological Medicine*, 27, 1205–1213.

Brown, G.W., Adler, Z., and Bifulco, A. (1988). Life events, difficulties and recovery from chronic depression. *British Journal of Psychiatry*, 153, 487–498.

Brugha, T.S. (ed.) (1995). *Social Support and Psychiatric Disorder: Research Findings and Guidelines for Clinical Practice*. Cambridge University Press, Cambridge UK.

Champion, L.A., Goodall, G., and Rutter, M. (1995). Behaviour problems in childhood and stressors in early adult life. I. A 20 year follow-up of London school children. *Psychological Medicine*, 25, 231–246.

Checkley, S.A., Slade, A.P., and Shur, E. (1981). Growth hormone and other responses to clonidine inpatients with endogenous depression. *British Journal of Psychiatry*, 138, 51–53.

Cohen, S. and Wills, T.A. (1985). Stress, social support and the buffering hypothesis. *Psychological Bulletin*, 98, 310–357.

Cole, M.G., Bellavance, F., and Mansour, A. (1999). Prognosis of depression in elderly community and primary care populations: a systematic review and meta-analysis. *American Journal of Psychiatry*, 156, 1182–1189.

Collier, D.A., Stober, G., Li, T., Heils, A., Catalano, M., Di Bella, D., *et al.* (1996). A novel functional polymorphism within the promoter of the serotonin transporter gene: possible role in susceptibility to affective disorders. *Molecular Psychiatry*, 1, 453–460.

Coryell, W., Endicott, J., Winokur, G., *et al.* (1995). Characteristics and significance of untreated major depressive disorder. *American Journal of Psychiatry*, 152, 1124–1129.

Coryell, W., Leon, A., Winokur, G., *et al.* (1996). Importance of psychotic features to long-term course in major depressive disorder. *American Journal of Psychiatry*, 153, 483–489.

Cowen, P.J. (1998). Pharmacological management of treatment-resistant depression. *Advances in Psychiatric Treatment*, 4, 320–327.

Davies, K.L., Davis, B.M., Mathé, A.A., Mohs, R.C., Rothpearl, A.B., Levy, M.I., Gorman, L.K., and Berger, P. (1984). Age and the dexamethasone suppression test in depresson. *American Journal of Psychiatry*, 141, 872–874.

Dawson, R., Lavori, P.W., Coryell, W.H., *et al.* (1998). Maintenance strategies for unipolar depression: an observational study of levels of treatment and recurrences. *Journal of Affective Disorders*, 49, 31–44.

Dikeos, D.G., Papadimitriou, G.N., Avramopoulos, D., *et al.* (1999). Association between the dopamine D3 receptor gene locus and unipolar affective disorders. *Psychiatric Genetics*, 9, 189–195.

DiMascio, A., Weissman, M., Prusoff, B., Neu, C., Zwilling, M., and Klerman, G. (1979). Differential symptom reduction by drugs and psychotherapy in acute depression. *Archives of General Psychiatry*, 36, 1451–1456.

Drevets, W.C., Price, J.L., Simpson, J.R., Jr, Todd, R.D., Reich, T., Vannier, M., and Raichle, M.E. (1997). Subgenual prefrontal cortex abnormalities in mood disorders. *Nature*, **386**, 824–827.

Elkin, I., Shea, M., Watkins, J., Imber, S., Sotsky, S., Collins, J., Glass, D., Pilkonis, P., Leber, W., Docherty, J., Fiester, S., and Parloff, M. (1992). National Institute of Mental Health treatment of depression collaborative treatment programme. *Archives of General Psychiatry*, **46**, 971–982.

Elliott, R., Sahakian, B.J., McKay, A.P., Herrod, J.J., Robbins, T.W., and Paykel, E.S. (1996). Neuropsychological impairments in unipolar depression: the influence of perceived failure on subsequent performance. *Psychological Medicine*, **26**, 975–989.

Elliott, R., Sahakian, B.J., Herrod, J.J., Robbins, T.W., and Paykel, E.S. (1997a). Abnormal response to negative feedback in unipolar depression: evidence for a diagnosis specific impairment. *Journal of Neurology, Neurosurgery and Psychiatry*, **63**(1), 74–82.

Elliott, R., Baker, S.C., Rogers, R.D., O'Leary, D.A., Paykel, E.S., Frith, C.D., Dolan, R.J., and Sahakian, B.J. (1997b). Prefrontal dysfunction in depressed patients performing a complex planning task: a study using positron emission tomography. *Psychological Medicine*, **27**, 931–942.

Elliott, R., Sahakian, B.J., Michael, A., Paykel, E.S., and Dolan, R.J. (1998). Abnormal neural response to feedback on planning and guessing tasks in patients with unipolar depression. *Psychological Medicine*, **28**, 559–571.

Emmerson, J.P., Burvill, P.W., Finlay-Jones, R., and Hall, W. (1989). Life events, life difficulties and confiding relationships in the depressed elderly. *British Journal of Psychiatry*, **155**, 787–792.

Farmer, A., Redman, K., Harris, T., Mahmood, A., Sadler, S., and McGuffin, P. (2001). Sensation-seeking, life events and depression. *British Journal of Psychiatry*, **178**, 549–552.

Fava, G.A., Grandi, S., Zielezny, M., Canestrari, R., and Morphy, M.A. (1994). Cognitive behavioural treatment of residual symptoms in primary major depressive disorder. *American Journal of Psychiatry*, **151**, 1295–1299.

Frank, E., Kupfer, D.J., Perel, J.M., Cornes, C., Jarrett, D.B., Maccinger, A.G., et al. (1990). Three year outcomes for maintenance therapies of recurrent depression. *Archives of General Psychiatry*, **47**, 1093–1099.

Frank, E., Prien, R.F., Jarrett, R.B., Keller, M.B., Kupfer, D.J., Lavori, P.W., Rush, A.J., and Weissman, M.M. (1991). Conceptualisation and rationale for consensus definitions of terms in major depressive disorder. Remission, recovery, relapse and recurrence. *Archives of General Psychiatry*, **48**, 851–855.

Gater, R.A., Dean, C., and Morris, J. (1989). The contribution of childbearing to the sex difference in first admission rates for affective psychosis. *Psychological Medicine*, **19**, 719–724.

Georgotas, A., McCue, R.E., and Cooper, T.B. (1989). A placebo-controlled comparison of nortriptyline and phenelzine in maintenance therapy of elderly depressed patients. *Archives of General Psychiatry*, **46**, 783–786.

Gottfries, C.G. (1998). Is there a difference between elderly and younger patients with regard to the symptomatology and aetiology of depression? *International Clinical Psychopharmacology*, **13** (Suppl. 5), 13–18.

Greenhouse, J.B., Kupfer, D.J., Frank, E., Jarrett, D.B., and Rejman, K.A. (1987). Analysis of time to stabilization in the treatment of depression: biological and clinical correlates. *Journal of Affective Disorders*, **28**, 1–9.

Greenwald, B.S., Kramer-Ginsberg, E., Bogerts, B., *et al.* (1997). Qualitative magnetic resonance imaging findings in geriatric depression. Possible link between later-onset depression and Alzheimer's disease. *Psychological Medicine*, **27**, 421–443.

Hagnell, O., Lanke, J., Rorsman, B., and Öjesjö, L. (1982). Are we entering an age of melancholy: Depressive illnesses in a prospective epidemiological study over 25 years: the Lundy Study, Sweden. *Psychological Medicine*, **12**, 279–289.

Hammen, C. (1991). Generation of stress in the course of unipolar depression. *Journal of Abnormal Psychology*, **100**, 555–561.

Harkness, K.L., Monroe, S.M., Simons, A.D., and Thase, M. (1999). The generation of life events in recurrent and non-recurrent depression. *Psychological Medicine*, **29**, 135–144.

Harris, E.C. and Barraclough, B. (1998). Excess mortality of mental disorder. *British Journal of Psychiatry*, **173**, 11–53.

Hein, C., Newport, D.J., Heit, S., Graham, Y.P., Wilcox, M., Bonsall, R., Miller, A.H., and Nemeroff, C.B. (2000). Pituitary-adrenal and autonomic responses to stress in women after sexual and physical abuse in childhood. *Journal of the American Medical Association*, **284**, 592–597.

Hermann, N., Lieff, S., and Silberfeld, M. (1989). The effect of age of onset on depression in the elderly. *Journal of Geriatric Psychiatry and Neurology*, **2**, 182–187.

Heuser, I., Yassouridis, A., and Holsboer, F. (1994). The combined dexamethasone. CRH test: a refined laboratory test for psychiatric disorders. *Journal of Psychiatric research*, **28**, 341–356.

Hunt, G.E., Johnson, G.F.S., and Caterson, I.D. (1989). The effect of age oncortisol and plasma dexamethasone concentrations in depressed patients and controls. *Journal of Affective Disorders*, **17**, 21–32.

Jarrett, R.B., Kraft, D., Doyle, J., Foster, B.M., Eaves, C.G., and Silver, P.C. (2001). Preventing recurrent depression using cognitive therapy with and without a continuation phase: a randomised clinical trial. *Archives of General Psychiatry*, **58**, 381–388.

Johnson, L., Andersson-Lundman, G., Åberg-Wistedt, A., and Mathé, A.A. (2000). Age of onset in affective disorder: its correlation with hereditary and psychosocial factors. *Journal of Affective Disorders*, **59**, 139–148.

Jorm, A.F. (1987). Sex and age differences in depression: a quantitative synthesis of published research. *Australian and New Zealand Journal of Psychiatry*, **21**, 46–53.

Jorm, A.F. (2000). Does old age reduce the risk of anxiety and depression? A review of epidemiological studies across the adult life span. *Psychological Medicine*, 30, 11–22.

Kaufmann, J., Plotsky, P.M., Nemeroff, C.B., and Charney, D.S. (2000). Effects of early adverse experiences onbrain structure and function: clinical implications. *Biological Psychiatry*, 48, 778–790.

Keller, M.B., Klerman, G.L., Lavori, P.W., Coryell, W., Endicott, J., and Taylor, J. (1984). Long-term outcome of episodes of major depression: clinical and public health significance. *Journal of the American Medical Association*, 252, 788–792.

Kendler, K.S. and Karkowski-Shuman, L. (1997). Stressful life events and genetic liability to major depression: genetic control of exposure to the environment? *Psychological Medicine*, 27, 539–547.

Kendler, K.S. and Prescott, C.A. (1999). A population-based twin study of lifetime major depression in men and women. *Archives of General Psychiatry*, 56, 39–44.

Kendler, K.S., Neale, M., Kessler, R., Heath, A., and Eaves, L. (1993). A twin study of recent life events and difficulties. *Archives of General Psychiatry*, 50, 789–796.

Kendler, K.S., Kessler, R.C., Walters, E.E., MacLean, C., Neale, M.C., Heath, A.C., and Eaves, L.J. (1995). Stressful life events, genetic liability, and onset of an episode of major depression in women. *American Journal of Psychiatry*, 152, 833–842.

Kendler, K.S., Karkowski, L.M., and Prescott, C.A. (1999a). Causal relationship between stressful life events and the onset of major depression. *American Journal of Psychiatry*, 156, 837–841.

Kendler, K.S., Karkowski, L.M., and Prescott, C.A. (1999b). The assessment of dependence in the study of stressful life events: validation using a twin design. *Psychological Medicine*, 29, 1455–1460.

Kendler, K.S., Thornton, L.M., and Gardner, C.O. (2000). Stressful life events and previous episodes in the etiology of major depression in women: an evaluation of the 'kindling' hypothesis. *American Journal of Psychiatry*, 157, 1243–1251.

Kienke, A.S. and Rosenbaum, J.F. (2000). Efficacy of venlafaxine in the treatment of severe depression. *Depression and Anxiety*, 12(Suppl. 1), 50–54.

Kiloh, L.G., Andrews, G.A., and Neilson, M. (1988). The long-term outcome of depressive illness. *British Journal of Psychiatry*, 153, 752–757.

Klein, D.N., Schatzberg, A.F., McCollough, J.P., et al. (1999). Age of onset in chronic major depression: relation to demographic and clinical variables, family history and treatment response. *Journal of Affective Disorders*, 55, 149–157.

Koenig, H.G. and Blazer, D.G. (1992). Epidemiology of geriatric affective disorders. *Clinics in Geriatric Medicine*, 8, 235–251.

Koenig, H.G., Cohen, H.J., Blazer, D.G., Krishnan, K.R.R., and Sibert, T. (1993). Profile of depressive symptoms in younger and older medical inpatients with major depression. *Journal of the American Geriatric Society*, 41, 1169–1176.

Lee, A.S. and Murray, R.M. (1988). The long-term outcome of Maudsley depressives. *British Journal of Psychiatry*, 153, 741–751.

Manki, H., Kanbe, S., Muramatsu, T., *et al.* (1996). Dopamine D2, D3 and D4 receptor and transporter gene polymorphisms and mood disorders. *Journal of Affective Disorders*, **40**, 7–13.

Mann, J.J., Huang, Y.Y., Underwood, M.D., *et al.* (2000). A serotonin transporter gene promoter polymorphism (5-HTTLPR) and prefrontal cortical binding in major depression and suicide. *Archives of General Psychiatry*, **57**, 729–738.

McGuffin, P., Kats, R., and Bebbington, P. (1988). The Camberwell Collaborative Depression Study. III. Depression and adversity in the relatives of depressed probands. *British Journal of Psychiatry*, **152**, 755–782.

Mervaala, E., Föhr, J., Könönen, M., Valkonen-Korhonen, M., Vainio, P., Partanen, K., Partanen, J., Tiihonen, J., Viinam:aki, H., Karjalainen, A.-K., and Lehtonen, J. (2000). Quantitative MRI of the hippocampus and amygdala in severe depression. *Psychological Medicine*, **30**, 117–125.

Methonen, O.P., Sogaard, J., Roponen, P., and Behnke, K. (2000). Randomized, double-blind comparison of venlafaxine and setraline in outpatients with major depressive disorder. Venlafaxine 631 Study Group. *Journal of Clinical Psychiatry*, **61**, 95–100.

Michael, A., Jenaway, A., Paykel, E.S., and Herbert, J. (2000). Altered salivary dehydroepiandrosterone levels in major depression in adults. *Biological Psychiatry*, **48**, 989–995.

Moore, P., Landolt, H.-P., Seifritz, E., Clark, C., Bhatti, T., Kelsoe, H., Rappaport, M., and Christian Gillin, J. (2000). Clinical and physiological consequences of rapid tryptophan depletion. *Neuropsychopharmacology*, **23**, 601–622.

Mueller, T.I., Leon, A.C., Keller, M.B., Solomon, D.A., Endocitt, J., Coryell, W., Warshaw, M., and Maser, J.D. (1999). Recurrence after recovery from major depressive disorder during 15 years of observational follow-up. *American Journal of Psychiatry*, **156**, 1000–1006.

Murphy, B.E.P. (1997). Antiglucocorticoid therapies in major depression: a review. *Psychoneuroendocrinology*, **22**(Suppl. 1), S125–S132.

Murphy, J.M., Laird, N.M., Monson, R.R., Sobol, A.M., and Leighton, A.H. (2000). Incidence of depression in the Stirling County Study: historical and comparative perspecctives. *Psychological Medicine*, **30**, 505–514.

Nelson, W.H., Orr, W.W., Shane, S.R., and Stevenson, J.M. (1984). Hypothalamic-pituitary-adrenal axis activity and age in major depression. *Journal of Clinical Psychiatry*, **45**, 120–121.

O'Brien, J., Ames, D., Chiu, E., Schweitzer, I., Desmond, P., and Tress, B. (1998). Severe deep white matter lesions and outcome in elderly patients with major depressive disorder: follow up study. *British Medical Journal*, **317**, 982–984.

O'Leary, D., Paykel, E.S., Todd, C., and Vardulaki, K. (2001). Suicide in primary affective disorders revisited: a systematic review by treatment era. *Journal of Clinical Psychiatry*, **62**, 804–811.

Ogilvie, A.D., Battersby, S., Bubb, V.J., *et al.* (1996). Polymorphism in serotonin transporter gene associated with suseptibility to major depression. *Lancet*, **347**, 731–733.

Old Age Depression Interest Group. (1993). How long should the elderly take antidepressants? A double blind placebo-controlled study of continuation/prophylaxis therapy with dothiepin. *British Journal of Psychiatry*, **162**, 175–182.

Ongur, D., Drevets, W.C., and Price, J.L. (1998). Glial reduction in the subgenual prefrontal cortex in mood disorders. Proceedings of the National Academy of Science, USA, Vol. 95, pp. 13290–13295.

Pande, A.C., Birkett, M., Fechner-Bates, S., Haskett, R.F., and Greden, J.F. (1996). Fluoxetine versus phenelzene in atypical depression. *Biological Psychiatry*, **40**, 1017–1020.

Park, S.B.G., Williamson, D.J., and Cowen, P.J. (1996). 5HT neuroendocrine function in major depression: prolactin andcortisol responses to D-fenfluramine. *Psychological Medicine*, **26**, 1191–1196.

Paykel, E.S. (1991). Depression in Women. *British Journal of Psychiatry*, **158**(10), 22–29.

Paykel, E.S. (1994*a*). Life events, social support and depression. *Acta Psychiatrica Scandinavica*, **89** (Suppl. 377), 50–58.

Paykel, E.S. (1994*b*). Psychological therapies. *Acta Psychiatrica Scandinavica, Dysthymia in Clinical Practice*, **89** (Suppl. 383), 35–41.

Paykel, E.S. (2000). Not an age of depression after all? Incidence rates may be stable over time. *Psychological Medicine*, **30**, 489–490.

Paykel, E.S. (2001*a*). Stress and affective disorders in humans. *Seminars in Clinical Neuropsychiatry*, **6**, 4–11.

Paykel, E.S. (2001*b*). Continuation and maintenance therapy in depression. *Brit Med Bull*, **57**, 145–159.

Paykel, E.S. and Cooper, Z. (1992). Life events and social stress. In E.S., Paykel (Ed.), *Handbook of Affective Disorders* (2nd edition) pp. 149–170.

Paykel, E.S., McGuinness, B.M., and Gomez, J. (1976). An Anglo-American comparison of the scaling of life events. *British Journal of Medical Psychology*, **49**, 237–247.

Paykel, E.S., Ramana, R., Cooper, Z., Hayhurst, H., Kerr, J., and Barocka, A. (1995). Residual symptoms after partial remission: an important outcome in depression. *Psychological Medicine*, **25**, 1171–1180.

Paykel, E.S., Cooper, Z., Ramana, R., and Hayhurst, H. (1996). Life events, social support and marital relationships in the outcome of severe depression. *Psychological Medicine*, **26**, 121–133.

Paykel, E.S., Scott, J., Teasdale, J.D., Johnson, A.L., Garland, A., Moore, R., Jenaway, A., Cornwall, P.L., Hayhurst, H., Abbott, R., and Pope, M. (1999). Prevention of relapse in residual depression by cognitive therapy. A controlled trial. *Arch. Gen. Psychiatry*, **56**, 829–835.

Paykel, E.S., Paykel, R., Abbott, R., Jenkins, T.S., Brugha, H., and Meltzer (2000). Urban-rural mental health differences in Great Britain: findings from the National Morbidity Survey. *Psychol. Med.*, **30**, 269–280.

Persson, M.L., Wasserman, D., Geijer, T., Jonsson, E.G., and Terenius, L. (1997). Tyrosine hydroxylase allelic distributionin suicide attempters. *Psychiatry Research*, **72**, 73–80.

Pfohl, B., Stangl, D., and Zimmerman, M. (1984). The implications of DSM-III personality disorders for patients with major depression. *Journal of Affective Disorders*, **7**, 309–318.

Phillips, K.A. and Nierenberg, A.A. (1994). The assessment and treatment of refractory depression. *Journal of Clinical Psychiatry*, **55** (Suppl.), 20–26.

Plomin, R., Lichtenstein, P., Pedersen, N., McClearn, G.E., and Nesselroade, J.R. (1990). Genetic influences on life events during the last half of the life span. *Psychology of Aging*, **5**, 25–30.

Poirier, M.F. and Boyer, P. (1999). Venlafaxine and paroxetine in treatment-resistant depression. Double-blind randomised comparison. *British Journal of Psychiatry*, **175**, 12–16.

Pollock, B.G., Ferrell, R.E., Mulsant, B.H., *et al.* (2000). Allelic variation in the serotonin transporter promoter affects onset of paroxetine treatment in late-life depression. *Neuropsychopharmacology*, **23**, 587–590.

Price, L.H., Carpenter, L.L., and Rasmussen, L.A. (2001). Drug combination strategies. In J.D., Amsterdam, M. Hornig, and A.A. Nierenberg (Eds.), *Treatment-Resistant Mood Disorders*, Cambridge University Press, Cambridge, United Kingdom, pp. 194–222.

Qian, Y., Lin, S., Jiang, S., Wu, X., Tang, G., and Wang, D. (1999). Studies of the DXS7 polymorphism at the MAO loci in unipolar depression. *American Journal of Medical Genetics*, **88**, 598–600.

Quitkin, F.M., Stewart, J.W., McGrath, P.J., *et al.* (1993). Colombia atypical depression. A subgroup of depressives with better response to MAOI than to tricyclic antidepressants or placebo. *British Journal of Psychiatry*, **163** (Suppl. 21), 30–34.

Ramana, R., Paykel, E.S., Cooper, Z., Hayhurst, H., Saxty, M., and Surtees, P.G. (1995). Remission and relapse in major depression: a two-year prospective follow-up study. *Psychological Medicine*, **25**, 1161–1170.

Ramana, R., Paykel, E.S., Surtees, P.G., Melzer, D., and Mehta, M. (1999). Medication received by patients with depression following the acute episode: adequacy and relation to outcome. *British Journal of Psychiatry*, **174**, 128–134.

Reimherr, F.W., Amsterdam, J.D., Quitkin, F.M., Rosenbaum, J.F., Fava, M., Zajecka, J., Beasley, C.M., Michelson, D., Roback, P., and Sundell, K. (1998). Optimal length of continuation therapy in depression: a prospective assessment during long-term fluoxetine treatment. *American Journal of Psychiatry*, **155**, 1247–1253.

Reynolds, C.F., Frank, E., Perel, J.M., Imber, S.D., Cornes, C., Miller, M.D., Maumdar, S., Houck, P.R., Dew, M.A., Stack, J.A., Pollock, B.G., and Kupfer, D.J. (1999). Nortriptyline and interpersonal psychotherapy as maintenance therapies for recurrent major depression: a randomised controlled trial in patients older than 59 years. *Journal of the American Medical Association*, **281**, 39–45.

Reynolds, C.F., III, Frank, E., Kupfer, D.J., *et al.* (1996). Treatment outcome in recurrent major depression: a post hoc comparison of elderly ('young old') and midlife patients. *American Journal of Psychiatry*, **153**, 1288–1292.

Ribeiro, S.C.M., Tandon, R., Grunhaus, L., and Greden, J.F. (1993). The DST as a predictor of outcome in depression: a meta-analysis. *American Journal of Psychiatry*, **150**, 1618–1229.

Robins, E. and Guze, S. (1972). Classification of affective disorders—the primary-secondary, the endogenenous-reactive and the neurotic-psychotic dichotomies. In T.A. Williams, M.M. Katz, and J.A. Shield (Eds.), *Recent Advances in Psychobiology of the Depressive Illnesses*, US Printing Office, Washington, pp. 283–293.

Roy-Byrne, P.P., Satng, P., Wittchen, H.-U., Ustun, B., Walters, E.E., and Kessler, R.C. (2000). Lifetime panic-depression comorbidity in the National Comorbidity Survey: association with symptoms, impairment, course and help-seeking. *British Journal of Psychiatry*, **176**, 229–235.

Rubinsztein, D.C., Leggo, J., Goodburn, S., Walsh, C., Jain, S., and Paykel, E.S. (1996). Genetic asociation between monoamine oxidase A microsatellite and RFLP alleles and bipolar affective disorder: analysis and meta-analysis. *Human Molecular Genetics*, **5**(6), 779–782.

Ryan, N.D., Puig-Antich, J., Ambrosini, P., *et al.* (1987). The clinical picture of major depression in children and adolescents. *Archives of General Psychiatry*, **44**, 854–861.

Schatzberg, A.F., Haddad, P., Kaplan, E.M., Lejoyex, M., Rosenbaum, J.F., Young, A.H., and Zajecka, J. (1997). Serotonin reuptake inhibitor discontinuation syndrome: a hypothetical definition. Discontinuation Consensus Panel. *Journal of Clinical Psychiatry*, **58**(Suppl. 7), 5–10.

Schulze, T.G., Muller, D.J., Krauss, H., *et al.* (2000). Association between a functional polymorphism in the monoamine oxidase A gene promoter and major depressive disorder. *American Journal of Medical Genetics*, **96**, 801–803.

Simpson, G.M., Lee, J.H., Cuculic, Z., and Kellner, R. (1976). Two doses of imipramine in hospitalized endogenous and neurotic depressives. *Archives of General Psychiatry*, **33**, 1093–1102.

Smith, A.L. and Weissman, M.M. (1992). Epidemiology. Chapter 8. In E.S. Paykel (Ed.), *Handbook of Affective Disorders*. (2nd edition) Churchill Livingstone, Edinburgh, pp. 111–129.

Stage, K.B., Bech, P., Kragh-Sørensen, P., Nair, N.P.V., Katona, C., and Danish University Antidepressant Group (2001). Differences in symptomatology and diagnostic profile in younger and elderly depressed inpatients. *Journal of Affective Disorders*, **64**, 239–248.

Sullivan, P.F., Neale, M.C., and Kendler, K.S. (2000). Genetic epidemiology of major depression: review and meta-analysis. *American Journal of Psychiatry*, **157**, 1552–1562.

Targum, S.D., Greenberg, R.D., Harmon, R.L., Kessler, K., Salerian, A.S., and Fram, D.H. (1984). Thyroid hormone and the TRH stimulation test in refractory depression. *Journal of Clinical Psychiatry*, **45**, 345–346.

Teasdale, J.D., Segal, Z.V., Williams, J.M., Ridgeway, V.A., Soulsby, J.M., and Lau, M.A. (2000). Prevention of relapse/recurrence in major depression by mindfulness-based cognitive therapy. *Journal of Consulting? Clinical Psychology*, **68**, 615–623.

Thase, M.E. and Rush, A.J. (1995). Treatment, 943–950.-resistant depression. In F.E. Bloom, and D.J., Kupfer (Eds.), *Psychopharmacology: The Fourth Generation of Progress*. Raven Press, New York, pp. 1081–1097.

Vaillant, G.E., Meyer, S.E., Mukamal, K., and Soldz, S. (1998). Are social supports inlate midlife a cause or a result of successful physical ageing? *Psychological Medicine*, **28**, 1159–1168.

van der Does, A.J.W. (2001). The effects of tryptophan depletion on mood and psychiatric symptoms. *Journal of Affective Disorders*, **64**, 107–119.

Van Os, J. and Jones, P. (1999). Developmental precursors of affective illness in a general population birth cohort. *Archives of General Psychiatry*, **54**, 625–631.

Wilcox, J.A., Ramirez, A.L., and Baida-Fragoso, N. (2000). The prognostic value of thought disorder in psychotic depression. *Annals of Clinical Psychiatry*, **12**, 1–4.

Young, W.P., Laws, E.R., Sharbrough, F.W., and Weinshilboum, R.M. (1986). Human monoaminoxidase: lack of brain and platelet correlation. *Archives of General Psychiatry*, **43**, 604–609.

Chapter 7

Later Life

John O'Brien and Alan Thomas

Introduction

Depression in late life remains a common condition. Snowdon (1990) observed that prevalence studies in late-life depression fall into two types: studies using recognized (usually DSM) diagnostic criteria, which yield rates of 1–3 per cent and studies assessing the presence of substantial depressive symptoms, which yield much higher rates of 10–16 per cent. These figures have been confirmed by the recent re-analysis of thirty-four community based epidemiological studies of depression in the elderly by the EURODEP consortium which found an average of 1.8 per cent for major depression and 13.5 per cent for all depressive syndromes (Beekman et al., 1999). Unlike dementia, which shows a clear association with increasing age, there is still some controversy over whether depression increases with age with the majority of studies showing that, if organic disorders such as dementia are excluded and disability controlled for, there is no change in prevalence with age (Jenkins et al., 1997; Roberts et al., 1997; Blazer, 1999). Females are still more likely to be affected than males, though this sex difference may narrow with increasing age (Jorm, 1987; Bebbington et al., 1998). The lack of association with ageing belies historic and psychoanalytical views that ageing itself was inherently depressogenic because of loss of youth and the fear of approaching death. Instead, while psychosocial factors still play a very important role, there is increasing evidence that biological factors have an important aetiological role, especially in those whose onset of affective disorder is in later life. This chapter will review clinical features, aetiology, treatment, and prognosis with this in mind.

Clinical features of late-life depression

Although the symptoms needed for the diagnosis of depression in the elderly are the same as those in younger adults, it has been suggested there may be a specific symptom profile characteristic of depression in the elderly. After reviewing the literature Baldwin (1994) concluded that overall there was little evidence for phenomenological differences between older and younger depressed patients. Certain features may be more characteristic of the elderly, but this is not necessarily due to depressive illness. For example, the concept of 'masked depression', in which elderly people complain of somatic problems and not low mood, has not generally been supported and the idea may have reflected a cohort effect; elderly people do not like to bother their doctor and may only do so for physical ailments (Baldwin, 1994). Two large studies addressing this have been conducted by Brodaty and colleagues (Brodaty *et al.*, 1991; Brodaty *et al.*, 1997). In their first study (Brodaty *et al.*, 1991) they examined 242 patients with DSM-III major depression, of whom sixty-one were aged sixty and over. This group of older patients was more severely depressed and had significantly more delusions, agitation, and appetite loss than the younger adults. In a later study Brodaty and colleagues (Brodaty *et al.*, 1997) examined 285 patients with DSM-III-R major depression and compared 208 younger patients (<60 years; mean age thirty-eight) with seventy-seven older patients (mean age sixty-nine). The older patients were again more severely depressed on standard rating scales and showed significantly more psychomotor disturbance and psychosis (both hallucinations and delusions), with such symptoms being rare in the younger group. Older patients also had more appetite loss, weight loss, somatic symptoms (hypochondriasis), and guilt. These studies, albeit from a tertiary mood disorders unit, suggest that psychosis, especially delusions, psychomotor disturbance, and appetite loss may be more common in the elderly.

Although neither of these studies by Brodaty and colleagues found a difference between early and late-onset depression, in their comparison of early and late onset depressed cases Baldwin and Tomenson (1995) found the former to have significantly more anxiety symptoms and borderline differences in agitation and somatic symptoms. Krishnan *et al.* (1995) carried out a larger study comparing elderly people with an early ($n = 113$) and late ($n = 113$) onset of their depression (cut-off age fifty). Severity of depression was similar in the two groups and the only symptom more common in the late onset group was apathy.

Cognitive impairment is a common feature of late-life depression although it is now recognized to be a common accompaniment of depression in all adults and arguably is part of the core of depressive illness (Austin *et al.*, 2001). Widespread impairments have been documented, especially in attention, memory and executive function. Deficits are probably more severe in elderly people with depression, especially those seen in hospital (Baldwin, 1994), though the extent to which this reflects modification by the presence of age-related changes is still debated. However, depression is now established as a risk factor for dementia (Jorm et al., 1991) and those who have severe cognitive impairments or 'pseudodementia' as part of their illness may be at highest risk (Kral and Emery, 1989).

In summary, the symptoms of depression remain the same in the elderly but there appears to be some change in their balance, at least in severely ill hospital subjects. Psychotic and psychomotor symptoms may be more common and cognitive impairments may occur more frequently. It is less clear whether people with an older age of onset of their depressive illness show a different balance of clinical features but they may show more apathy and less anxiety.

Aetiological factors

Family history

Current evidence indicates that genetic risk is reduced in people whose first episode of depression is in later life. Hopkinson (1964) examined 100 successive hospital patients over the age of fifty with 'manic depression' and compared them with ninety-nine first-degree relatives. Patients with a first episode before fifty were compared with a later onset group. Twenty per cent of relatives of early onset patients had had an affective illness compared with only 8 per cent for the late onset group. Similar findings have been reported by others (Mendlewicz, 1976; Baldwin and Tomenson, 1995) and Brodaty and colleagues found 29 per cent of early onset patients had a family history of affective disorder compared with only 13 per cent of the late onset patients (Brodaty et al., 1991). These studies certainly suggest that genetic factors make less of a contribution to the aetiology of late-life depression.

Life events, social support, and physical Illness

Murphy (1982) studied 119 elderly (over sixty-five) depressed subjects and 168 community controls matched for age and sex. She found severe independent life-events, for example, bereavement, life threatening illness to someone close and financial/material loss, were much more common in the depressed patients in the year before the depression; 48 per cent of the depressed subjects had suffered severe events compared with 23 per cent of the controls. The largest difference was in severe illness to the subject but other differences were significant even when this was left out of the analysis. Consistent with this, chronic poor health (over two years) was also significantly more common in the depressed elderly, occurring in 39 per cent compared with 26 per cent of controls. Major social difficulties (again over two years and severe) were also associated with increased depression; 42 per cent in the depressed subjects compared with 19 per cent in the controls. Lack of a confiding relationship ('intimacy') was found to be a vulnerability factor to depression in the elderly. These findings are similar to those of Brown and Harris (1978) in younger women. Emmerson *et al.* (1989) conducted a similar study in Perth in which they compared 101 elderly depressed subjects (age >60) with eighty-five community controls. They also found that severe life events were associated with depression, though only when occurring in the previous three months, and that lack of a close confidant also increased the risk of depression but only in men. There was no difference between the groups in the frequency of non-severe events or general life difficulties.

Prince and colleagues (Prince *et al.*, 1997*a,b*, 1998) conducted a community-based study of 654 elderly people in the Gospel Oak district of London. Using a very broad definition of depression they found a prevalence rate of 17 per cent, with depression associated with female gender, living alone, low income and low social support but the strongest association was with disability and handicap. They also found associations with life events such as bereavement, personal illness, and theft, especially when these occurred in the preceding six months (Prince *et al.*, 1997*b*). In a subsequent, prospective, study disablement (especially handicap), loneliness, lack of social support, divorce or separation (plus marriage for women only), and a range of physical health problems (especially sleep disturbance, pain, and breathlessness) were all associated with incident depression (Prince *et al.*, 1997*b*). Schoevers *et al.* (2000*a*) conducted a three-year prospective study in Amsterdam examining the risk factors for incident depression in a large ($n = 4051$) community cohort. Sixteen per cent developed a depressive episode over a 3-year period with personal history of depression, disability, chronic disease, and loss of spouse again found to be risk factors.

In summary, severe independent life events (bereavement, life threatening illness, to someone close, severe personal illness, and financial losses) in the months preceding depression appear to be risk factors and loneliness/ lack of a confidant seems to be a vulnerability factor for depression in elderly people. Whilst chronic ill health and associated disability/handicap are also linked with increases in depressive symptoms it is not clear they lead to an increase in the syndrome of major depression.

Biological factors

Abnormalities in the hypothalamic-pituitary-adrenal (HPA) axis including raised cortisol levels, non-suppression on the dexamethasone suppression test (DST), CRH hypersecretion, enhanced adrenal response to ACTH and pituitary, and adrenal hypertrophy have been associated with depression regardless of age (O'Brien *et al.*, 1993). However, HPA axis abnormalities have been strongly associated with advancing age in most studies with elderly subjects showing the highest rates of DST non-suppression and the greatest cortisol levels (O'Brien *et al.*, 1993). If such changes are indeed aetiologically related to depressed mood, as has been postulated, then HPA axis activation is likely to play a much more important role in aetiology of depression in the elderly than at other ages. There may be a particular relationship between HPA axis activation and cognitive impairments which is discussed in detail later. However, other biological factors may also play an important role in the aetiology of late life depression. The association of physical illness and disability with depressive symptoms raises the question of whether any particular type of illness may be more relevant. The most likely location for disease processes to affect mood is, of course, the brain and cerebral organic disorders such as Alzheimer's disease, vascular dementia, stroke, dementia with Lewy bodies, and Parkinson's disease have very high rates of depression (20–40 per cent) (Pohjasvaara *et al.*, 1998; Ballard *et al.*, 1999; Ballard *et al.*, 2000; Cummings, 1992). There is increasing evidence of a close link between depression in the elderly, particularly late-onset depression, and vascular disease in general and cerebrovascular disease in particular which will now be discussed.

Vascular disease and depression

Depression and coronary artery disease

The earliest studies suggesting a link between psychological profile and vascular disease did not study depression but the so-called 'type A' personality (highly competitive, driven, and time pressured) (Jenkins, 1976*a*,*b*). Subsequently, studies have demonstrated coronary artery disease (CAD) to be associated with increased rates of depression and poorer outcome. Frasure-Smith *et al.* (1993) studied 222 post-infarct patients and found 16 per cent with modified DSM- III-R major depression between days 5 and ten in hospital. In a study of 200 patients, undergoing cardiac catheterization and coronary angiography, Hance *et al.* (1996) found 17 per cent had major depression and the same percentage had 'minor depression'. Hippisley-Cox *et al.* (1998) conducted a large case-control study in a general practise population and found 20 per cent of those with CAD to have depression compared with 12 per cent of the controls. Large community studies have also shown that depression predicts subsequent development of cardiovascular disease in both younger (Pratt *et al.*, 1996; Ford *et al.*, 1998) and older populations (Ariyo *et al.*, 2000; Penninx *et al.*, 2001). For example, Ford *et al.* followed up 1190 men (medical students) for forty years as part of the Johns Hopkins Precursors Study (Ford *et al.*, 1998). Over the follow-up period the cumulative incidence of depression was 12 per cent (those with depression at baseline were excluded) and they found this group had a significant increase in coronary artery disease (RR 2.12 (1.24–3.63)) and myocardial infarction (MI)(RR 2.12 (1.11–4.06)) compared with their non-depressed peers. The depressive episode preceded the heart disease by a median of fifteen years.

The presence of depression in those with CAD is associated with a poor prognosis. Frasure-Smith *et al.* (1993) showed that, even controlling for other prognostic factors, depression was an important predictor of poor outcome after MI, increasing mortality three and a half times at six months, making it as strong a predictor of poor outcome as the best established risk factor, left ventricular dysfunction. They followed up these subjects to eighteen months (Frasure-Smith *et al.*, 1995) and found major depression continued to significantly predict a similar increased mortality.

There are four main mechanisms by which depression could plausibly increase the risk of subsequent vascular disease. The first is by psychosocial mechanisms such as increasing the likelihood of smoking (Breslau *et al.*, 1998). Second is HPA axis dysfunction, since administered steroids have long been known to lead to high levels of circulating cholesterol and triglycerides as well as hypertension and Troxler *et al.* (1977) demonstrated high cortisol levels to be correlated with the severity of coronary atherosclerosis. Third would be via platelet and clotting changes which could in turn link to the atherogenic process as several studies have shown depression to be associated with platelet activation, clotting abnormalities and an increase in inflammatory cytokines (Musselman *et al.*, 1996; Laghrissi-Thode *et al.*, 1997; Connor and Leonard, 1998). Finally a mechanism that may be related to the increased mortality in depressed subjects with CAD is reduced heart rate variability. This puts subjects at increased risk of arrhythmias and is an independent predictor of increased mortality in CAD (Musselman *et al.*, 1998). Carney *et al.* (1995) found heart rate variability was significantly reduced in depressed patients with CAD compared to non-depressed patients. Antidepressant treatment is unlikely to be a confounder as, if anything, cardiovascular mortality was even higher in subjects before the introduction of antidepressants (Weeke *et al.*, 1987) while the Epidemiological Catchment Area Study in the United States found no effect of antidepressants on cardiovascular mortality (Pratt *et al.*, 1996). Furthermore, Sauer *et al.* (2001) have reported a case-control study of middle-aged adults comparing cardiovascular mortality in 653 depressed subjects and 2990 controls. After adjustment for relevant risk factors they found treatment with selective serotonin reuptake inhibitors (SSRI's) was associated with a significant reduction in MI (OR 0.35; 95 per cent CI 0.18–0.68) compared to non-users but that other antidepressant drug classes showed no such reduction. Thus, there is no reason depression in those with CAD should not be vigorously treated, with SSRIs being the treatment of choice; indeed treating depression after MI may improve prognosis.

In summary, a large body of research suggests a bi-directional link between depression and CAD. Thus depression itself seems to be a significant risk factor for the subsequent development of CAD and MI and those with pre-existing CAD have a high prevalence of depression which predicts poor cardiovascular outcome.

Depression and cerebrovascular disease

Emotional incontinence and depression both have strong associations with cerebrovascular disease. Robinson *et al.* (1983) examined 103 consecutive stroke patients at Johns Hopkins in Baltimore and found 27 per cent met criteria for major depression and nearly 50 per cent had some depressive syndrome in the immediate post-stroke period (first two weeks). Subsequent studies have confirmed that depression after stroke is clearly increased with an incidence of 15–30 per cent for major depression and 20–40 per cent if minor depression is included (Morris *et al.*, 1990; House *et al.*, 1991; Andersen *et al.*, 1994; Burvill *et al.*, 1995; House, 1996; Pohjasvaara *et al.*, 1998; Rao, 2000). For example, a well-conducted Finnish stroke study of 277 consecutive stroke patients assessed 3–4 months after stroke found major depression in 26 per cent and minor depression in 14 per cent (Pohjasvaara *et al.*, 1998). Several prospective studies, mainly in the elderly, have shown that, as with CAD, depression is itself predictive of future stroke and is associated with an increased risk of between 50 and 150 per cent (Colantonio *et al.*, 1992; Simonsick *et al.*, 1995; Wassertheil-Smoller *et al.*, 1996; Everson *et al.*, 1998; Jonas and Mussolino, 2000). Taken together these studies show depression is an independent risk factor for stroke and indicate that, like CAD, stroke has a close bi-directional relationship with depression in which each may be a risk factor for the other.

There remains controversy over the importance of lesion location as a predictor of the development of depression. The initial study of Robinson and colleagues (Robinson and Szetela, 1981) compared eighteen subjects after a left hemispheric stroke with eleven subjects with a traumatic brain injury and found a correlation between proximity of the stroke lesion to the frontal pole and depressive symptoms. While that group has repeated this observation (Robinson *et al.*, 1985; Morris *et al.*, 1996), others have found an association with right sided stroke (MacHale *et al.*, 1998) and some have reported no association at all (Gonzalez-Torrecillas *et al.*, 1995). A recent comprehensive review concluded that the issue was still unclear (Carson *et al.*, 2000).

Although depression has long been associated with vascular dementia, for example, it is a diagnostic feature incorporated into Hackinski's 1974 ischaemic scale (Hachinski *et al.*, 1975), there have been few well-conducted studies in this area. However, reports based on both hospital and community cohorts have reported higher prevalences of depression in vascular dementia (20–30 per cent) than in Alzheimer's disease (10–20 per cent) (Reding *et al.*, 1985; Cummings *et al.*, 1987; Reichman and Coyne, 1995; Ballard *et al.*, 2000), again suggesting an association between cerebrovascular disease and depression.

Vascular risk factors and depression

Depression has also been associated with vascular risk factors. A link with hypertension has been proposed (Rabkin *et al.*, 1983), though not all studies support this and a link with hypotension has also been suggested (Paterniti *et al.*, 2000). As such, the relationship between hypertension and depression is unclear at present. A stronger association has been shown with diabetes (Gavard *et al.*, 1993) identified nine cross-sectional studies investigating the relationship between depression and diabetes mellitus. All included a comparison group of non-diabetics. Four of the studies used structured clinical interviews to diagnose major depression and they found a mean prevalence of major depression of 14 per cent in adults with diabetes, which was significantly more than in the comparison subjects in three of the studies. The other five studies used depression rating scales and found a rate of all types of depression of 32 per cent; this was significantly greater than the comparison groups in all five studies. This finding appeared to apply to both type I and type II diabetes.

One important prospective study has addressed the issue of whether depression precedes or follows the development of diabetes. Eaton *et al.* (1996) used data from the Epidemiologic Catchment Area study in East Baltimore and found that major depression at baseline predicted an increased risk of developing diabetes of about twofold, although this just missed statistical significance. While further evidence is needed it remains possible that depression may not only be a consequence of diabetes but, as for CAD and stroke, actually be a risk factor for its subsequent development. Some community studies have found a link between low cholesterol and depression, for instance Morgan *et al.* (1993) found that men over seventy (but not younger men) with a low cholesterol (<4.14 mmol/l) had a threefold increase in depression. However, confounding factors such as weight loss and poor nutrition may be important and others have suggested that the relationship disappears once these are taken into account (Brown *et al.*, 1994). In a large statin trial cholesterol lowering (by 27 per cent) was not associated with an increase in depression (Wardle *et al.*, 1996). In summary, despite a plausible mechanism by which low cholesterol may cause a reduction in serotonergic receptors, no clear link with depression has emerged.

Overall, findings suggest a strong bi-directional link between depression and both cerebrovascular and cardiovascular disease. There is a link between diabetes and depression but no clear relationship between depression and other vascular risk factors has yet emerged.

Neuroimaging changes and depression

Many neuroimaging studies have demonstrated a range of abnormalities in elderly depressed subjects compared with matched controls. Jacoby and Levy conducted the first computed tomography (CT) study in affective disorders (Jacoby and Levy, 1980). They scanned forty-two subjects with affective disorder and fifty controls and found patients had larger ventricles. This was particularly the case for those with a late onset of depression. Since then a large number of CT and later magnetic resonance imaging (MRI) studies in depression at all ages have been conducted. These were reviewed by Soares and Mann (1997) who concluded that although many studies have found evidence of cerebral atrophy, ventricular dilatation, and sulcal enlargement in depression others have not and that the only consistent findings in depression are smaller frontal lobes and basal ganglia and an increase in signal hyperintensities in the white matter, especially in the frontal lobes. White matter hyperintensities may be periventricular, when they are associated with ventricular enlargement and ependymal changes, or in the deep white matter, where they are often associated with arteriosclerosis. Most studies have shown that it is deep white matter, rather than periventricular, lesions which are associated with depression. Coffey *et al.* (1993) reported a 7 per cent reduction in frontal lobe volume in depression and both their group and others have identified that an increase in white matter and subcortical grey matter hyperintensities is strongly associated with depression, especially late-onset depression (Coffey *et al.*, 1990; Greenwald *et al.*, 1996; O'Brien *et al.*, 1996a; Greenwald *et al.*, 1998). Iidaka *et al.* (1996) examined thirty elderly depressives matched for age, sex and vascular risk factors, and thirty controls. They reported an association of basal ganglia lesions, pontine lesions, and frontal white matter lesions with depression. Similarly Greenwald *et al.* (1996) studied forty-eight elderly depressives and thirty-nine healthy elderly subjects and found an association between basal ganglia lesions and depression. In a later study the same group (Greenwald *et al.*, 1998) scanned thirty-five elderly depressives and thirty-one controls and found location of hyperintensities in the left putamen and left frontal deep white matter showed significant associations with depression. These studies suggest that hyperintensities in the white matter of the frontal lobes and basal ganglia might have associations with major depression in the elderly. O'Brien and colleagues found a clear relationship with age of onset, with 50 per cent of late-onset (first episode after age sixty-five) cases having severe white matter change compared to under 20 per cent for similarly aged patients who had early onset depression (O'Brien *et al.*, 1996a).

While most studies have been of hospitalized patients, two large community studies have now confirmed the relationship between deep white matter lesions and depression in general and, in particular, late-onset depression. The first enrolled subjects from the Cardiovascular Health Study, which had participants from four major centres in the United States. A sample of 3660 elderly subjects (over sixty-five years) was obtained who had had both an MRI scan and complete depression data. Severity of white matter change and severity of basal ganglia lesions were both significantly associated with depression score but after adjusting for confounders only the link with basal ganglia lesions and depression remained significant (Steffens *et al.*, 1999). The Rotterdam Scan Study (de Groot *et al.*, 2000) recruited 1077 subjects aged sixty to ninety years from two large cohort studies in Rotterdam and Zoetermeer. Cognitively impaired subjects were excluded. Although basal ganglia lesions were not examined, the presence of lesions was associated with depression and someone with severe white matter change had a three to fivefold increase in the likelihood of having depression. Severe deep white matter lesions were associated with a late onset (over sixty years) of depression.

There is increasing evidence that such lesions are associated with treatment resistance and poor outcome. In a study of thirty-nine selected subjects from a tertiary service Hickie *et al.* (1995) found that white matter lesions significantly predicted poorer global clinical outcome after ECT or pharmacotherapy at sixteen weeks and poor global functioning, development of a probable dementia syndrome and institutionalization at one year (Hickie *et al.*, 1996). Simpson and colleagues (Simpson *et al.*, 1997; Simpson *et al.*, 1998) examined response to treatment and outcome in a more representative group of elderly depressives, who were drawn from consecutive referrals to consultant psychiatrists in Manchester. They found that lesions in the white matter of the frontal lobes, the basal ganglia and the pontine reticular formation predicted poor outcome to pharmacotherapy but not to ECT. The latter could be related to the relatively small numbers (sixteen) in this group but the authors plausibly argue it suggests ECT could be a more appropriate treatment for elderly depressed subjects with white matter lesions. O'Brien *et al.* (1998) carried out the longest follow-up study to date of fifty-four out of sixty elderly depressed subjects assessed for MRI hyperintensities (O'Brien *et al.*, 1996a). Severe deep white matter change was significantly associated with poor outcome, with none of the thirteen patients with severe change being continuously well over the follow-up period (mean thirty-two months).

The anatomic location of these findings is important because specific neural circuitry, reciprocally linking frontal cortical areas to the basal ganglia (the frontal-subcortical circuits, FSC) has for several years frequently been proposed as the likely site for any cerebral pathology to produce depression (Buchsbaum *et al.*, 1986; Cummings, 1993a,b; Mayberg *et al.*, 1994; Austin and Mitchell, 1995; Soares and Mann, 1997). There are far fewer functional imaging studies in elderly subjects with depression but those which have been reported suggest predominantly frontal (dorsolateral prefrontal cortex and anterior cingulate cortex) and basal ganglia changes (Bench *et al.*, 1993; Awata *et al.*, 1998; Tutus *et al.*, 1998; Halloran *et al.*, 1999), some of which which may reverse on recovery from illness (Bench *et al.*, 1995; Halloran *et al.*, 1999). Overall, such studies provide support, albeit limited, for fronto-striatal dysfunction in elderly subjects with depression.

Vascular depression

These studies show that white matter lesions, predominantly affecting fronto-striatal areas, are associated with depression in the elderly, particularly late-onset depression, and these lesions predict treatment resistance and poor outcome. Together with the strong link between vascular, especially cerebrovascular, disease, and depression such evidence has led to the 'vascular depression' hypothesis that vascular damage to key FSC plays an important role in the aetiology of late-life depression (Alexopoulos *et al.*, 1997a). As this is largely based on studies showing associations and imaging findings it raises the question as to whether there is direct neuropathological evidence to support this. It is only recently that this issue has been addressed. Using material (twenty depressed cases and twenty age-matched controls) from the Newcastle brain bank we have conducted a series of studies showing an increase in atheromatous disease at post-mortem in depressed cases

(Thomas *et al.*, 2001) and an increase in inflammatory markers associated with ischaemia (intracellular adhesion molecule-1 (ICAM-1) and vascular adhesions molecule (VCAM), most particularly in dorsolateral prefrontal cortex (Thomas *et al.*, 2000). We have subsequently undertaken post-mortem MRI and examined lesions detected radiologically to determine their anatomical location and their aetiology (Thomas *et al.*, 2002). Strikingly, depressed cases were associated with a highly significant increase in ischaemic as opposed to non-ischaemic lesions and such lesions were particularly found in dorsolateral prefrontal cortex. Such findings strongly support the vascular depression hypothesis of late-life depression and suggest dorsolateral prefrontal cortex as an important anatomical site where pathology predisposes to depression.

It is less clear whether such 'vascular' cases are different clinically from 'non-vascular' cases. Alexopoulos *et al.* (1997*a*), who first coined the term 'vascular depression', studied sixty-five elderly depressed subjects and found those with 'vascular depression' (defined on the basis of having one or more vascular risk factors) had a later age of onset, more severe psychomotor retardation, poorer insight, more cognitive impairment (especially frontal-executive impairment) but less depressive ideation, guilt, and agitation. Krishnan *et al.* (1997) examined eighty-nine people with major depression and used the presence of moderate to severe white matter change on MRI to divide the group into vascular (thirty-seven subjects) and non-vascular (fifty-two) groups. Those with 'vascular depression' were older, had a later age of onset and were less frequently psychotic. Vascular depressives also less frequently had a family history of depression. The clinical features suggested by Alexopoulos *et al.* (1997*b*) were not supported but Krishnan's study also did not find group differences in clinical vascular factors (rated in a manner which appears similar to that of Alexopoulos) either. The inconsistency here probably relates in part to the likely heterogeneity in the aetiology of depression but the main problem is the two studies used completely different methods for classifying 'vascular depression'. Similarly, in a large study of vascular risk factors and depression in the elderly no clear increase in risk factors could be demonstrated (Lyness *et al.*, 1998). In their MRI study O'Brien *et al.* attempted to control for vascular risk factors and still found a significant increase in white matter changes in the depressed group (O'Brien *et al.*, 1996*a*). These studies suggest that unravelling the contribution of vascular pathology to depression will not be easy, since depressed subjects may be more likely to suffer vascular damage (as evidenced by white matter lesions and manifest as depression) for a given burden of known vascular risk factors. Genetic susceptibility may be one reason and a recent report of a polymorphism in a gene which may be involved with regulating homocysteine levels is of interest in this regard (Hickie *et al.*, 2001).

Cognitive impairments and late-life depression

Frequency and profile of deficits

The occurrence of severe cognitive deficits in elderly patients with depression has long been recognized and the clinical importance of not misdiagnosing 'pseudodementia' as dementia has often been highlighted (Wells, 1979; McAllister, 1983). However, the relationship between depression and cognitive impairments is complex as many, if not all, elderly depressed subjects have subtle impairments on cognitive tasks if tested using sophisticated tests. Moreover, cognitive deficits are not always reversible on recovery of mood while depression is an established risk factor for Alzheimer's disease with an odds ratio of around (Jorm *et al.*, 1991).

In an important and detailed early study of cognitive dysfunction in elderly depression Abas *et al.* (1990) examined twenty patients with major depression, comparing them with twenty controls and nineteen patients with probable Alzheimer's disease. Depressed subjects had significant impairments in measures of attention, memory, and learning compared to the controls and about 70 per cent of the depressed group showed significant dysfunction on a test of new learning when depressed. Surprisingly, the pattern was similar to that in the Alzheimer's group although the depressed subjects were less severely affected. When recovered, although the depressed patients improved they remained significantly impaired and slowed compared to controls.

The same group later went on to assess executive function in a different group of twenty-four depressed cases (Beats *et al.*, 1996), finding significant deficits on tests of attentional shifting, spatial planning, and spatial working memory. Deficits were less severe than those found in frontal-subcortical disorders, for example, Parkinson's disease and Huntington's disease. On recovery there was some improvement but deficits persisted in simple and choice reaction times, perseveration, and verbal fluency. Others have reported a very similar profile of neuropsychological impairments with some, but incomplete, improvement on recovery from depression (Dahabra *et al.*, 1998). In summary, elderly patients with depression have marked impairments on a wide range of tests including attention, memory and learning, and executive function which may persist despite clinical recovery. The three main possibilities for explaining such deficits, neurotransmitter disturbances, HPA axis dysfunction and structural brain changes, will now be examined.

Neurotransmitter disturbances

Many neurotransmitters which may be involved in the genesis of depression, such as serotonin, noradrenaline, and dopamine, also play an important role in cognition. The transmitter most implicated in current theories of depression is serotonin. It is possible to manipulate serotonergic levels using the technique of acute tryptophan depletion (ATD) whereby an amino acid load (given as a drink) causes a marked (70 per cent+) but transient lowering of blood and brain tryptophan, and serotonin. Cognitive impairments after ATD have been described in normal controls and in patients with Alzheimer's disease (Park *et al.*, 1994; Porter *et al.*, 2000). We have recently used this technique in a study of elderly depressed subjects and shown significant impairments in global cognitive function, new learning, and some aspects of executive function (unpublished results). Such effects on cognition appear independent of an effect on mood. However, ATD does not appear to mimic either the full profile or the severity of cognitive deficits seen during depression and the continuing deficits despite clinical recovery would argue against transmitter change as the sole cause of impairments.

HPA axis dysfunction

Another possibility is HPA axis dysfunction and, in particular, the raised cortisol levels which occur during depression. Raised cortisol levels are, of course, a prominent feature of depression at all ages but dysregulation of the axis occurs as a part of normal ageing and there is a particularly strong and robust relationship between hypercortisolaemia during depression and advancing age, such that elderly depressed subjects have the most marked increases and the highest rates of DST non-suppression (O'Brien *et al.*, 1993; O'Brien *et al.*, 1996*b*). The deleterious effects of prolonged and raised steroid levels have long been recognized. For example, Cushing's syndrome is associated with cognitive impairments, ventricular enlargement, and hippocampal atrophy (Starkman *et al.*, 1992) with prospective studies showing reversal of hippocampal changes and memory impairments once the Cushing's has been treated and cortisol levels return to normal (Starkman *et al.*, 1999).

Evidence suggesting important links between cortisol, cognition and brain changes has been reviewed in detail by (Sapolsky *et al.*, 1986; Sapolsky and Plotsky, 1990; Sapolsky, 2000). Essentially, animal studies have clearly shown that prolonged exposure to glucocorticoids can have adverse effects on the hippocampus. The hippocampus is an important site of glucocorticoid action, containing the highest concentration of the two receptor types (mineralocorticoid and glucocorticoid) of any brain area (McEwen and Sapolsky, 1995). Stimulation of these receptors mediates negative feedback while their loss leads to disinhibition of the axis. During ageing there is a gradual rise in glucocorticoid levels associated with hippocampal cell loss, with clear evidence the two are aetiologically related (Sapolsky, 2000). For example, adrenalectomy with low dose steroid replacement abolishes the normal hippocampal cell loss during ageing (Landfield et al., 1981). Raised steroid levels are toxic to hippocampal neurones, causing initially reduced dendritic sprouting and subsequently cell death by increasing calcium influx and/or disrupting cell energy metabolism (Landfield and Eldridge, 1994). A link with ageing is suggested by the finding that it is the hippocampus of older, not younger, animals which is most susceptible to the neurotoxic effects of cortisol. Prolonged stress in primates has also been associated with marked hippocampal cell loss (Uno et al., 1989). A number of studies in volunteer subjects and in the healthy elderly do give support for the view that raised cortisol levels, either during stress or after exogenous cortisol administration, can cause impairments in declarative memory (Kirschbaum et al., 1996). This is clearly an important area for study, since antiglucocorticoid treatments are available and could potentially be used to treat cognitive dysfunction in elderly subjects with depression. Since the hippocampus is an important site of cognitive function, particularly for new learning and memory, might cognitive impairments during depression in the elderly be due to hypercortisolaemia and subsequent hippocampal dysfunction and/or damage?

Despite the convincing background support for this hypothesis, direct evidence of this as an important mechanism in humans is still required. Depression has been associated with hippocampal volume reduction in some studies, indeed in one study the degree of volume reduction was inversely correlated with duration of depression providing indirect support for a toxic effect of cortisol (Sheline et al., 1999). However, there have been contradictory studies and the largest study to date of hippocampal volume in elderly depressed subjects showed no reduction (Ashtari et al., 1999). Moreover, hippocampal volume reductions have been found in many other psychiatric diseases including schizophrenia and post-traumatic stress disorder where links with prolonged hypercortisolaemia are less clear. The only study to report a correlation between raised cortisol during depression and reduced hippocampal volume (Axelson et al., 1993) was in younger subjects whose hippocampal volume was actually no different to controls. Many, though by no means all, studies have found an association between cognitive impairments and raised cortisol levels, though the effects of age may be an important confounder in such studies. However, these studies often find the association is not only limited to memory tasks, but also which might be expected if hippocampal damage alone were the explanation.

In summary, a convincing case can be made that raised cortisol levels might induce cognitive impairments through hippocampal damage in elderly depressed subjects, though there has not yet been a clear demonstration that glucocorticoid mediated hippocampal damage definitely occurs. While further studies are needed to address this important issue it should be remembered there are other mechanisms which may explain a relationship between cortisol and cognitive impairments, one of which is the effects of cortisol in impairing serotonergic function (McAllister-Williams *et al.*, 1998).

Structural brain changes

These have been suggested by several groups as important factors underlying cognitive impairments, particularly for white matter lesions on MRI. Salloway *et al.* (1996) examined thirty elderly subjects divided into early and late-onset groups (cut-off age sixty). The late-onset group had significantly more periventricular and deep white matter lesions on MRI and were more impaired on executive and verbal and non-verbal memory tasks. Similarly, Lesser *et al.* (1996) examined a large group of controls ($n = 165$) and early ($n = 35$) and late ($n = 65$) onset depressed cases (using age fifty). Depressed subjects as a groups scored significantly worse than controls on measures of executive function, non-verbal memory and non-verbal intelligence. There was also evidence for an association between poor executive function and burden of white matter change on MRI. In a study of executive dysfunction and white matter change depressed subjects showed worse performance globally than controls but were specifically impaired on tests of attention, frontal lobe function, and general memory (Kramer-Ginsberg *et al.*, 1999). Those with moderate-to-severe deep white matter lesions performed significantly worse than both depressed subjects without such lesions and controls; no such interactions were found for periventricular hyperintensities or subcortical grey matter hyperintensities. In contrast, a small but carefully conducted study of nineteen recovered elderly depressed subjects and fourteen controls failed to find an association between significant impairments in verbal memory and slowed reaction times and burden of white matter change on MRI (Dahabra *et al.*, 1998). However, subjects had a relatively young age (mean sixty-six) and lacked power because of small numbers.

Interestingly, cognitive dysfunction, particularly executive dysfunction, has been associated with poor clinical outcome (Simpson *et al.*, 1998; Alexopoulos *et al.*, 2000). Alexopoulos *et al.* (2000) assessed patients every two weeks during the continuation phase and monthly during the maintenance phase of a placebo-controlled treatment trial of nortriptyline. Initiation/perseveration scores derived from the Mattis dementia scale, but not memory scores, were found to predict relapse in the continuation phase. Forty-three patients then agreed to participate in the maintenance phase and again impairment in initiation/perseveration but not memory predicted recurrence. Although MRI findings were not available in this group, it is tempting to speculate that severe white matter change, which has been linked with both executive dysfunction and poor outcome, may be the substrate underlying this association.

Taken together all these studies highlight the importance of a frontal-subcortical pattern of attentional and executive impairments in depression in addition to memory deficits and suggest white matter changes may explain some of the reasons for this. One difficulty is that studies have not usually controlled for age (in that both executive dysfunction and white matter changes appear more common in older subjects, and specifically those with late-onset depression). Such changes would explain impairments continue on recovery but not why significant improvement occurs with recovery of mood, since lesions with such a structural basis are unlikely to alter.

Conclusion

It is clear that cognitive impairments in elderly patients with depression are frequent, may be severe, and affect a wide range of domains including attention, memory, and executive function. Despite a number of studies, investigating transmitter changes, HPA axis dysfunction and structural brain changes as possible causes, the underlying aetiology is still unclear and likely to be multifactorial. Improvements in cognitive function are seen on recovery and reverses in transmitter abnormalities and cortisol levels may be important in this regard. Structural brain changes may be important in explaining the continuing deficits which occur despite clinical recovery, the two most likely candidates being hippocampal changes (which may be caused or exacerbated by hypercortisolaemia) and white matter lesions, presumably due to ischaemia. However, the time course of development of these changes, their progression or otherwise over time and the extent to which they explain the intriguing finding that depression is a risk factor for subsequent Alzheimer's disease requires further study. Only long term prospective studies combining serial cognitive, endocrine, and brain imaging studies with post-mortem neuropathological examination will be able to provide answers to these clinically important questions.

Treatment and outcome

Naturalistic outcome of depression

Over the years various researchers have commented on the high mortality amongst elderly patients with depression and their generally poor prognosis. This bleak outlook was confirmed by a metaanalysis by Cole and Bellavance of elderly people (mean age over sixty) with depression managed in the community, mainly by primary care services (Cole *et al.*, 1999). They examined twelve outcome studies up to 1996 which met their quality criteria, involving a total of 1268 patients. At two years after the index episode of depression they found 33 per cent were well, 33 per cent were still depressed and 21 per cent were dead. The rest were classified as 'other' and seemed to represent a poor outcome group since they included those who developed dementia and had only partial remissions. They observed that although most of the studies had weaknesses, the two largest and best executed studies had very similar findings (Kennedy *et al.*, 1991; Copeland *et al.*, 1992). Similar conclusions were reached by the same authors in another metaanalysis of elderly medical inpatients with depression (Cole and Bellavance, 1997*a*). Data from eight studies on 265 patients revealed that at three months only 18 per cent were rated as well whilst 43 per cent were still depressed and 22 per cent were dead. By twelve months only 19 per cent were well, 29 per cent still depressed and 53 per cent had died. However, it is encouraging that the best outcome was found in a third metaanalysis of people with late-life depression who were seen by hospital psychiatric services (Cole and Bellavance, 1997*b*). This analysis of 1487 patients in sixteen studies who had all been followed for at least a year found 60 per cent were either well or had relapses with good recovery, 14–22 per cent were continuously ill with the remainder again having poor outcomes such as death (ranging from 3 to 19 per cent dead by twelve months) or developing dementia. Again although many of the studies were regarded as having weaknesses the overall findings are close to those of the larger and better executed studies in the analysis (Baldwin and Jolley, 1986; Burvill *et al.*, 1991; Baldwin *et al.*, 1993). The high mortality in medical inpatients is not surprising but the poorer outcome in community psychiatric patients is counter-intuitive as they have less severe depressive illness and might therefore be expected to have a better outcome than those people seen as inpatients. The reason is probably the sad reality of under detection and under treatment, with Cole reporting a figure of only 20 per cent of elderly depressed people in the community receiving adequate treatment (Cole *et al.*, 1999) and Sharma (Sharma *et al.*, 1998) giving a figure of 10 per cent.

Treatment

A number of randomized controlled trials have clearly demonstrated that antidepressant treatment improves short term outcome compared to placebo in elderly patients with depression. A recent Cochrane review identified seventeen randomized controlled studies and found convincing evidence for tricyclic antidepressants, SSRI's and monoamine oxidase inhibitors over six weeks (Wilson *et al.*, 2001). Studies by Reynolds and colleagues in older subjects have also demonstrated an excellent response to antidepressants in older subjects, at least equivalent to younger subjects, though longer treatment (8–10 weeks rather than six) may sometime be needed (Reynolds *et al.*, 1996). There is also good evidence to support the widely held clinical view that ECT is at least as effective in treating elderly people with depression as the young. Tew *et al.* (1999) compared the efficacy of ECT in 268 subjects split into three age groups: the 'old old' (over seventy-five); the 'young old' (60–74) and younger adults (under sixty). Improvements in depression were (non-significantly) greatest in the two older age-groups with no differences in adverse events.

There is not as much evidence regarding the effects of maintenance treatment in the elderly. The first study to address this compared 75 mg dothiepin with placebo over a two year period in those who had recovered from a major depressive episode (Anonymous, 1993). Dothiepin treatment reduced relapse rates by 2.5-fold. A similar study of nortriptyline found relapse rates of 50 per cent in those switched to placebo and 20 per cent in those maintained on active treatment (Alexopoulos *et al.*, 2000).

In a well conducted three year study Reynolds and colleagues compared antidepressant (nortriptyline) treatment, inter-personal therapy, their combination and placebo in the prevention of recurrence of depression (Reynolds *et al.*, 1999b). All active treatments were better than placebo, with combined treatment being the most efficacious. Whilst providing important support for long term maintenance treatment in the elderly this study also highlighted the efficacy of psychological treatments, helping to counter the often expressed but erroneous view that the elderly are unable to benefit from psychological treatments.

Such studies indicate that the elderly can have good response to anti-depressant treatments and ECT, though they may require slightly longer treatment period to recover. Meats *et al.* (1991) undertook one of the few studies attempting to examine the effects of age on outcome by directly comparing younger and older depressed subjects treated as in-patients by the same clinical team. They found elderly subjects did just as well as younger patients. Others have shown that although initial short term response to antidepressant treatment is similar regardless of age, older patients may have higher relapse rates (Reynolds *et al.*, 1999*a*) and the influence of cerebral white matter changes on outcome may be relevant in this regard. Overall, there is every reason to be optimistic regarding therapeutic response in older subjects though they may take longer to respond and be more in need of longer term maintenance therapy.

Increased mortality

The classic study of Murphy *et al.* (1988) highlighted the increased mortality in elderly depressed subjects treated within secondary care, with a threefold increase compared to a control group. A number of recent prospective studies have tried to examine whether depression is an independent factor for this increase or whether it is due to confounding variables. Pulska *et al.* (1999) examined the outcome of 813 subjects examined in 1984 and 1989 in Finland. They found 48 per cent of those depressed at each time point had died compared with only 26 per cent who were never depressed, a highly significant increase. Those depressed only at baseline (31 per cent dead) did not differ significantly from those who were never depressed. Penninx and colleagues in Amsterdam followed a cohort of 3056 subjects (mean age seventy) over 4 years (Penninx *et al.*, 1999). Major depression ($n = 61$, 2 per cent) was determined by DSM-III criteria and they also defined a group with minor depression ($n = 392$, 13 per cent). For minor depression they found men but not women had a significant 1.80-fold increase in all cause mortality but that for major depression both sexes had a significant 1.83-fold increase in mortality. The same group (Schoevers *et al.*, 2000*b*) reported similar findings in another cohort of 4051 elderly subjects living in the community in Amsterdam who were followed over 6 years. At baseline 13 per cent of the subjects were rated as having a depression (based on GMS), with 11 per cent rated as neurotic (approximating minor depression) and 2 per cent 'psychotic' (approximating major depression). Survival analysis showed only men with 'neurotic' depression had a significant increase in mortality of 1.67-fold whilst both men and women with 'psychotic' depression had significant increases in mortality of about 2-fold. Finally Schulz and colleagues examined 5201 subjects over sixty-five (mean age seventy-three) in four centres in the United States (Schulz *et al.*, 2000). Depression was assessed using a modified 10-item CES-D at baseline and 20 per cent met their cut-off criteria for depression. Subjects were followed over 6 years and those with baseline depression had a 24 per cent increase in mortality. This figure was obtained after extensive controlling in the analyses for all important sociodemographic and physical illness risk factors; the other three prospective studies controlled for most but not all such factors.

In summary these studies uniformly confirm the high mortality associated with late-life depression, whether it is major or minor depression, and suggest men may have higher depression related mortality. They show that depression itself is clearly an independent risk factor for this increased mortality. However, the strong association between depression and vas-cular diseases is very relevant as in most studies cardiovascular and cerebrovascular disease account for a substantial proportion of this increased mortality. Another possible link would be carcinoma, since depression is frequently associated with cancer and may sometimes be the first manifestation.

Prognostic factors

There is a surprising lack of agreement over factors which may influence outcome. Studies have not reported any consistent differences in outcome due to sex or age, once other confounders such as severity of depression and physical illness have been controlled for. Greater severity of initial depression was reported by Murphy (1983) to predict poorer outcome but other studies have found no such association (Baldwin and Jolley, 1986; Burvill *et al.*, 1991). Similarly Murphy (1983) found illness for twelve months before treatment predicted a worse outcome but Baldwin and Jolley did not find duration of illness predicted outcome (Baldwin and Jolley, 1986). Again Murphy (1983) found the occurrence of adverse life events following the onset of depression had a particularly adverse effect on outcome but Burvill *et al.* (1991) found no such relationship. Physical ill-health (Murphy, 1983; Baldwin and Jolley, 1986; Burvill *et al.*, 1991; Cole and Bellavance, 1997*b*) and cognitive impairment (Cole and Bellavance, 1997*b*) have, unsurprisingly, been found to be associated with a worse outcome, with the latter being associated particularly with an increased risk of dementia (Jorm, 2000). The only other consistent predictors of outcome appear to be the cerebral factors already discussed, a higher burden of white matter lesions being associated with poor response to treatment and increased mortality (Hickie *et al.*, 1995; Simpson *et al.*, 1997; O'Brien *et al.*, 1998) and prefrontal dysfunction, probably also due to cerebrovascular disease, predicting poor treatment response and increased relapse and recurrence (Kalayam and Alexopoulos, 1999; Alexopoulos *et al.*, 2000).

Conclusions

Depression in late life remains common and although the symptom profile is similar to that at younger ages the elderly tend to present with more melancholia, psychosis, and cognitive impairments which may persist despite subsequent recovery. The relative contributions of various putative aetiologic factors remains to be precisely defined but adverse life events and social isolation remain important while concurrent physical ill-health and subtle organic cerebral factors that may relate to vascular disease are implicated, particularly in those whose first depression occurs in late life. The aged brain may be particularly susceptible to the deleterious effects of hypercortisolaemia, though whether HPA axis abnormalities during depression contribute to permanent structural brain changes remains unclear. Standard antidepressant therapies including antidepressant drugs, psychological treatments, and ECT are effective in the elderly, though a longer period of treatment may be required. Such therapies are also effective in preventing relapse, at least over periods up to three years, which is particularly relevant because of the high relapse rates seen in untreated patients. Longer term outcome is poor in naturalistic studies but much improved in treated patients. A high (2–3 fold increase) mortality is evident, while depression remains an important risk factor for subsequent dementia. All these factors highlight the need for careful detection of depression in later life combined with vigorous treatment and careful follow-up to monitor maintenance treatment and the progression of symptoms such as cognitive dysfunction.

Acknowledgements

We thank the Wellcome Trust and the Stanley Foundation for financial support.

References

Baldwin, R.C. (1994). Is there a distinct type of major depression in the elderly? *Journal of Psychopharmacology*, **8**, 177–184.

Blazer, D. (1999). EURODEP consortium and late-life depression. *British Journal of Psychiatry*, **174**, 284–285.

Cummings, J.L. (1992). Depression and Parkinson's disease: a review. *American Journal of Psychiatry*, **149**, 443–454.

Cummings, J.L. (1993a). Frontal-subcortical circuits and human behavior. *Archives of Neurology*, **50**, 873–880.

Cummings, J.L. (1993b). The neuroanatomy of depression. *Journal of Clinical Psychiatry*, **54**, 14–20.

Hopkinson, G. (1964). A genetic study of affective illness in patients over 50. *British Journal of Psychiatry*, **110**, 244–254.

House, A. (1996). Depression associated with stroke. *Journal of Neuropsychiatry and Clinical Neurosciences*, **8**, 453–457.

Jenkins, C.D. (1976a). Medical progress. Recent evidence supporting psychologic and social risk factors for coronary disease (first of two parts). *New England Journal of Medicine*, **294**, 987–994.

Jenkins, C.D. (1976b). Recent evidence supporting psychologic and social risk factors for coronary disease. *New England Journal of Medicine*, **294**, 1033–1038.

Jorm, A.F. (1987). Sex and age differences in depression: a quantitative synthesis of published research. *Australian & New Zealand Journal of Psychiatry*, **21**, 46–53.

Jorm, A.F. (2000). Is depression a risk factor for dementia or cognitive decline? A review. *Gerontology*, **46**, 219–227.

Mendlewicz, J. (1976). The age factor in depressive illness: some genetic considerations. *Journal of Gerontology*, **31**, 300–303.

Murphy, E. (1982). Social origins of depression in old age. *British Journal of Psychiatry*, **141**, 135–142.

Murphy, E. (1983). The prognosis of depression in old age. *British Journal of Psychiatry*, **142**, 111–119.

Rao, R. (2000). Cerebrovascular disease and late life depression: an age old association revisited. *International Journal of Geriatric Psychiatry*, **15**, 419–433.

Snowdon, J. (1990). The prevalence of depression in old Age. *International Journal of Geriatric Psychiatry*, **5**, 141–144.

Austin, M.P. and Mitchell, P. (1995). The anatomy of melancholia: does frontal-subcortical pathophysiology underpin its psychomotor and cognitive manifestations? *Psychological Medicine*, **25**, 665–672.

Baldwin, R.C. and Jolley, D.J. (1986). The prognosis of depression in old age. *British Journal of Psychiatry*, **149**, 574–583.

Baldwin, R.C. and Tomenson, B. (1995). Depression in later life. A comparison of symptoms and risk factors in early and late onset cases. *British Journal of Psychiatry*, **167**, 649–652.

Brown, G.W. and Harris, T.O. (1978). *Social Origins of Depression*. Tavistock, London.

Cole, M.G. and Bellavance, F. (1997a). Depression in elderly medical inpatients: a meta-analysis of outcomes. *Cmaj*, **157**, 1055–1060.

Cole, M.G. and Bellavance, F. (1997b). The prognosis of depression in old age. *American Journal of Geriatric Psychiatry*, **5**, 4–14.

Connor, T.J. and Leonard, B.E. (1998). Depression, stress and immunological activation: the role of cytokines in depressive disorders. *Life Sciences*, **62**, 583–606.

Jacoby, R.J. and Levy, R. (1980). Computed tomography in the elderly. 3. Affective disorder. *British Journal of Psychiatry*, **136**, 270–275.

Jonas, B.S. and Mussolino, M.E. (2000). Symptoms of depression as a prospective risk factor for stroke. *Psychosomatic Medicine*, **62**, 463–471.

Kalayam, B. and Alexopoulos, G.S. (1999). Prefrontal dysfunction and treatment response in geriatric depression. *Archives of General Psychiatry*, **56**, 713–718.

Kral, V.A. and Emery, O.B. (1989). Long-term follow-up of depressive pseudodementia of the aged. *Canadian Journal of Psychiatry – Revue Canadienne de Psychiatrie*, **34**, 445–446.

Reichman, W.E. and Coyne, A.C. (1995). Depressive symptoms in Alzheimer's disease and multi-infarct dementia. *Journal of Geriatric Psychiatry and Neurology*, **8**, 96–99.

Robinson, R.G. and Szetela, B. (1981). Mood change following left hemispheric brain injury. *Annals of Neurology*, **9**, 447–453.

Soares, J.C. and Mann, J.J. (1997). The anatomy of mood disorders—review of structural neuroimaging studies. *Biological Psychiatry*, **41**, 86–106.

Abas, M.A., Sahakian, B.J., and Levy, R. (1990). Neuropsychological deficits and CT scan changes in elderly depressives. *Psychological Medicine*, **20**, 507–520.

Alexopoulos, G.S., Meyers, B.S., Young, R.C., Campbell, S., Silbersweig, D., and Charlson, M. (1997*a*). 'Vascular depression' hypothesis. *Archives of General Psychiatry*, **54**, 915–922.

Alexopoulos, G.S., Meyers, B.S., Young, R.C., Kakuma, T., Silbersweig, D., and Charlson, M. (1997*b*). Clinically defined vascular depression. *American Journal of Psychiatry*, **154**, 562–565.

Alexopoulos, G.S., Meyers, B.S., Young, R.C., *et al.* (2000). Executive dysfunction and long-term outcomes of geriatric depression. *Archives of General Psychiatry*, **57**, 285–290.

Andersen, G., Vestergaard, K., Riis, J., and Lauritzen, L. (1994). Incidence of post-stroke depression during the first year in a large unselected stroke population determined using a valid standardized rating scale. *Acta Psychiatrica Scandinavica*, **90**, 190–195.

Anonymous. (1993). How long should the elderly take antidepressants? A double-blind placebo-controlled study of continuation/prophylaxis therapy with dothiepin. Old Age Depression Interest Group. *British Journal of Psychiatry*, **162**, 175–182.

Ariyo, A.A., Haan, M., Tangen, C.M., *et al.* (2000). Depressive symptoms and risks of coronary heart disease and mortality in elderly Americans. Cardiovascular Health Study Collaborative Research Group. *Circulation*, **102**, 1773–1779.

Ashtari, M., Greenwald, B.S., Kramer-Ginsberg, E., *et al.* (1999). Hippocampal/amygdala volumes in geriatric depression. *Psychological Medicine*, **29**, 629–638.

Austin, M.P., Mitchell, P., and Goodwin, G.M. (2001). Cognitive deficits in depression: possible implications for functional neuropathology. *British Journal of Psychiatry*, **178**, 200–206.

Awata, S., Ito, H., Konno, M., *et al.* (1998). Regional cerebral blood flow abnormalities in late-life depression: relation to refractoriness and chronification. *Psychiatry & Clinical Neurosciences*, **52**, 97–105.

Axelson, D.A., Doraiswamy, P.M., McDonald, W.M., *et al.* (1993). Hypercortisolaemia and hippocampal changes in depression. *Psychiatry Research*, **47**, 163–173.

Baldwin, R.C., Benbow, S.M., Marriott, A., Tomenson, B. (1993). Depression in old age. A reconsideration of cerebral disease in relation to outcome. *British Journal of Psychiatry*, **163**, 82–90.

Ballard, C., Holmes, C., McKeith, I., *et al.* (1999). Psychiatric morbidity in dementia with lewy bodies: a prospective clinical and neuropathological comparative study with Alzheimer's disease. *American Journal of Psychiatry*, **156**, 1039–1045.

Ballard, C., Neill, D., O'Brien, J., McKeith, I.G., Ince, P., and Perry, R. (2000). Anxiety, depression and psychosis in vascular dementia: prevalence and associations. *Journal of Affective Disorders*, **59**, 97–106.

Beats, B.C., Sahakian, B.J., and Levy, R. (1996). Cognitive performance in tests sensitive to frontal lobe dysfunction in the elderly depressed. *Psychological Medicine*, **26**, 591–603.

Bebbington, P.E., Dunn, G., Jenkins, R., *et al.* (1998). The influence of age and sex on the prevalence of depressive conditions: report from the National Survey of Psychiatric. *Psychological Medicine*, **28**, 9–19.

Beekman, A.T.F., Copeland, J.R.M., and Prince, M.J. (1999). Review of community prevalence of depression in later life. *British Journal of Psychiatry*, **174**, 307–311.

Bench, C.J., Frackowiak, R.S., and Dolan, R.J. (1995). Changes in regional cerebral blood flow on recovery from depression. *Psychological Medicine*, **25**, 247–261.

Bench, C.J., Friston, K.J., Brown, R.G., Frackowiak, R.S., and Dolan, R.J. (1993). Regional cerebral blood flow in depression measured by positron emission tomography: the relationship with clinical dimensions. *Psychological Medicine*, **23**, 579–590.

Breslau, N., Peterson, E.L., Schultz, L.R., Chilcoat, H.D., and Andreski, P. (1998). Major depression and stages of smoking. A longitudinal investigation. *Archives of General Psychiatry*, **55**, 161–166.

Brodaty, H., Luscombe, G., Parker, G., *et al.* (1997). Increased rate of psychosis and psychomotor change in depression with age. *Psychological Medicine*, **27**, 1205–1213.

Brodaty, H., Peters, K., Boyce, P., *et al.* (1991). Age and depression. *Journal of Affective Disorders*, **23**, 137–149.

Brown, S.L., Salive, M.E., Harris, T.B., Simonsick, E.M., Guralnik, J.M., and Kohout, F.J. (1994). Low cholesterol concentrations and severe depressive symptoms in elderly people. *Bmj*, **308**, 1328–1332.

Buchsbaum, M.S., Wu, J., DeLisi, L.E., *et al.* (1986). Frontal cortex and basal ganglia metabolic rates assessed by positron emission tomography with [18F] 2-deoxyglucose in affective illness. *Journal of Affective Disorders*, **10**, 137–152.

Burvill, P.W., Hall, W.D., Stampfer, H.G., and Emmerson, J.P. (1991). The prognosis of depression in old age. *British Journal of Psychiatry*, **158**, 64–71.

Burvill, P.W., Johnson, G.A., Jamrozik, K.D., Anderson, C.S., Stewart-Wynne, E.G., and Chakera, T.M. (1995). Prevalence of depression after stroke: the Perth Community Stroke Study. *British Journal of Psychiatry*, **166**, 320–327.

Carney, R.M., Saunders, R.D., Freedland, K.E., Stein, P., Rich, M.W., and Jaffe, A.S. (1995). Association of depression with reduced heart rate variability in coronary artery disease. *American Journal of Cardiology*, **76**, 562–564.

Carson, A.J., MacHale, S., Allen, K., *et al.* (2000). Depression after stroke and lesion location: a systematic review. *Lancet*, **356**, 122–126.

Coffey, C.E., Figiel, G.S., Djang, W.T., and Weiner, R.D. (1990). Subcortical hyperintensity on magnetic resonance imaging: a comparison of normal and depressed elderly subjects. *American Journal of Psychiatry*, **147**, 187–189.

Coffey, C.E., Wilkinson, W.E., Weiner, R.D., *et al.* (1993). Quantitative cerebral anatomy in depression. A controlled magnetic resonance imaging study. *Archives of General Psychiatry*, **50**, 7–16.

Colantonio, A., Kasi, S.V., and Ostfeld, A.M. (1992). Depressive symptoms and other psychosocial factors as predictors of stroke in the elderly. *American Journal of Epidemiology*, **136**, 884–894.

Cole, M.G., Bellavance, F., and Mansour, A. (1999). Prognosis of depression in elderly community and primary care populations: a systematic review and meta-analysis. *American Journal of Psychiatry*, **156**, 1182–1189.

Copeland, J.R., Davidson, I.A., Dewey, M.E., *et al.* (1992). Alzheimer's disease, other dementias, depression and pseudodementia: prevalence, incidence and three-year outcome in Liverpool. *British Journal of Psychiatry*, **161**, 230–239.

Cummings, J.L., Miller, B., Hill, M.A., and Neshkes, R. (1987). Neuropsychiatric aspects of multi-infarct dementia and dementia of the Alzheimer type. *Archives of Neurology*, **44**, 389–393.

Dahabra, S., Ashton, C.H., Bahrainian, M., *et al.* (1998). Structural and functional abnormalities in elderly patients clinically recovered from early- and late-onset depression. *Biological Psychiatry*, **44**, 34–46.

de Groot, J.C., de Leeuw, F., Oudkirk, M., Hofman, A., Jolles, J., and Breteler, M.B. (2000). Cerebral white matter lesions and depressive symptoms in elderly adults. *Archives of General Psychiatry*, **57**, 1071–1076.

Eaton, W.W., Armenian, H., Gallo, J., Pratt, L., and Ford, D.E. (1996). Depression and risk for onset of type II diabetes. A prospective population-based study. *Diabetes Care*, **19**, 1097–102.

Emmerson, J.P., Burvill, P.W., Finlay-Jones, R., and Hall, W. (1989). Life events, life difficulties and confiding relationships in the depressed elderly. *British Journal of Psychiatry*, **155**, 787–792.

Everson, S.A., Roberts, R.E., Goldberg, D.E., and Kaplan, G.A. (1998). Depressive symptoms and increased risk of stroke mortality over a 29-year period. *Archives of Internal Medicine*, **158**, 1133–1138.

Ford, D.E., Mead, L.A., Chang, P.P., Cooper-Patrick, L., Wang, N.Y., and Klag, M.J. (1998). Depression is a risk factor for coronary artery disease in men: the precursors study. *Archives of Internal Medicine*, **158**, 1422–1426.

Frasure-Smith, N., Lesperance, F., and Talajic, M. (1993). Depression following myocardial infarction. Impact on 6-month survival. *Jama*, **270**, 1819–1825.

Frasure-Smith, N., Lesperance, F., and Talajic, M. (1995). Depression and 18-month prognosis after myocardial infarction. *Circulation*, **91**, 999–1005.

Gavard, J.A., Lustman, P.J., and Clouse, R.E. (1993). Prevalence of depression in adults with diabetes. An epidemiological evaluation. *Diabetes Care*, **16**, 1167–1178.

Gonzalez-Torrecillas, J.L., Mendlewicz, J., and Lobo, A. (1995). Effects of early treatment of poststroke depression on neuropsychological rehabilitation. *International Psychogeriatrics*, **7**, 547–560.

Greenwald, B.S., Kramer-Ginsberg, E., Krishnan, K.R., Ashtari, M., Auerbach, C., and Patel, M. (1998). Neuroanatomic localization of magnetic resonance imaging signal hyperintensities in geriatric depression. *Stroke*, **29**, 613–617.

Greenwald, B.S., Kramer-Ginsberg, E., Krishnan, R.R., Ashtari, M., Aupperle, P.M., and Patel, M. (1996). MRI signal hyperintensities in geriatric depression. *American Journal of Psychiatry*, **153**, 1212–1215.

Hachinski, V.C., Iliff, L.D., Zilhka, E., *et al.* (1975). Cerebral blood flow in dementia. *Archives of Neurology*, **32**, 632–637.

Halloran, E., Prentice, N., Murray, C.L., *et al.* (1999). Follow-up study of depression in the elderly. Clinical and SPECT data. *British Journal of Psychiatry*, **175**, 252–258.

Hance, M., Carney, R.M., Freedland, K.E., and Skala, J. (1996). Depression in patients with coronary heart disease. A 12-month follow-up. *General Hospital Psychiatry*, **18**, 61–65.

Hickie, I., Scott, E., Mitchell, P., Wilhelm, K., Austin, M.P., and Bennett, B. (1995). Subcortical hyperintensities on magnetic resonance imaging: clinical correlates and prognostic significance in patients with severe depression. *Biological Psychiatry*, **37**, 151–160.

Hickie, I., Scott, E., Naismith, S., *et al.* (2001). Late-onset depression: genetic, vascular and clinical contributions. *Psychological Medicine*, **31**, 1403–1412.

Hickie, I., Scott, E., Wilhelm, K., and Brodaty, H. (1996). Subcortical hyperintensities on magnetic resonance imaging in patients with severe depression-a longitudinal evaluation. *Biological Psychiatry*, **42**, 367–374.

Hippisley-Cox, J., Fielding, K., and Pringle, M. (1998). Depression as a risk factor for ischaemic heart disease in men: population based case-control study. *Bmj*, **316**, 1714–1719.

House, A., Dennis, M., Mogridge, L., Warlow, C., Hawton, K., and Jones, L. (1991). Mood disorders in the year after first stroke. *British Journal of Psychiatry*, **158**, 83–92.

Iidaka, T., Nakajima, T., Kawamoto, K., *et al.* (1996). Signal hyperintensities on brain magnetic resonance imaging in elderly depressed patients. *European Neurology*, **36**, 293–299.

Jenkins, R., Lewis, G., Bebbington, P., *et al.* (1997). The National Psychiatric Morbidity surveys of Great Britain—initial findings from the household survey. *Psychological Medicine*, **27**, 775–789.

Jorm, A.F., van Duijn, C.M., Chandra, V., *et al.* (1991). Psychiatric history and related exposures as risk factors for Alzheimer's zdisease: a collaborative re-analysis of case-control studies. EURODEM Risk Factors Research Group. *International Journal of Epidemiology*, **20**, S43–47.

Kennedy, G.J., Kelman, H.R., and Thomas, C. (1991). Persistence and remission of depressive symptoms in late life. *American Journal of Psychiatry*, **148**, 174–178.

Kirschbaum, C., Wolf, O.T., May, M., Wippich, W., and Hellhammer, D.H. (1996). Stress- and treatment-induced elevations of cortisol levels associated with impaired declarative memory in healthy adults. *Life Sciences*, **58**, 1475–1483.

Kramer-Ginsberg, E., Greenwald, B.S., Krishnan, K.R., *et al.* (1999). Neuropsychological functioning and MRI signal hyperintensities in geriatric depression. *American Journal of Psychiatry*, **156**, 438–444.

Krishnan, K.R., Hays, J.C., and Blazer, D.G. (1997). MRI-defined vascular depression. *American Journal of Psychiatry*, **154**, 497–501.

Krishnan, K.R., Hays, J.C., Tupler, L.A., George, L.K., and Blazer, D.G. (1995). Clinical and phenomenological comparisons of late-onset and early-onset depression. *American Journal of Psychiatry*, **152**, 785–788.

Laghrissi-Thode, F., Wagner, W.R., Pollock, B.G., Johnson, P.C., and Finkel, M.S. (1997). Elevated platelet factor 4 and beta-thromboglobulin plasma levels in depressed patients with ischemic heart disease. *Biological Psychiatry*, **42**, 290–295.

Landfield, P.W., Baskin, R.K., and Pitler, T.A. (1981). Brain aging correlates: retardation by hormonal-pharmacological treatments. *Science*, **214**, 581–584.

Landfield, P.W. and Eldridge, J.C. (1994). Evolving aspects of the glucocorticoid hypothesis of brain aging: hormonal modulation of neuronal calcium homeostasis. *Neurobiology of Aging*, **15**, 579–588.

Lesser, I.M., Boone, K.B., Mehringer, C.M., Wohl, M.A., Miller, B.L., and Berman, N.G. (1996). Cognition and white matter hyperintensities in older depressed patients. *American Journal of Psychiatry*, **153**, 1280–1287.

Lyness, J.M., Caine, E.D., Cox, C., King, D.A., Conwell, Y., and Olivares, T. (1998). Cerebrovascular risk factors and later-life major depression. Testing a small-vessel brain disease model. *American Journal of Geriatric Psychiatry*, **6**, 5–13.

MacHale, S.M., O'Rourke, S.J., Wardlaw, J.M., and Dennis, M.S. (1998). Depression and its relation to lesion location after stroke. *Journal of Neurology, Neurosurgery & Psychiatry*, **64**, 371–374.

Mayberg, H.S., Lewis, P.J., Regenold, W., and Wagner, H.N., Jr. (1994). Paralimbic hypoperfusion in unipolar depression. *Journal of Nuclear Medicine*, **35**, 929–934.

McAllister, T.W. (1983). Overview: pseudodementia. *American Journal of Psychiatry*, **140**, 528–533.

McAllister-Williams, R.H., Ferrier, I.N., and Young, A.H. (1998). Mood and neuropsychological function in depression: the role of corticosteroids and serotonin. *Psychological Medicine*, **28**, 573–584.

McEwen, B.S. and Sapolsky, R.M. (1995). Stress and cognitive function. *Current Opinion in Neurobiology*, **5**, 205–216.

Meats, P., Timol, M., and Jolley, D. (1991). Prognosis of depression in the elderly. *British Journal of Psychiatry*, **159**, 659–663.

Morgan, R.E., Palinkas, L.A., Barrett-Connor E.L., and Wingard, D.L. (1993). Plasma cholesterol and depressive symptoms in older men. *Lancet*, **341**, 75–79.

Morris, P.L., Robinson, R.G., and Raphael, B. (1990). Prevalence and course of depressive disorders in hospitalized stroke patients. *International Journal of Psychiatry in Medicine*, **20**, 349–364.

Morris, P.L., Robinson, R.G., Raphael, B., and Hopwood, M.J. (1996). Lesion location and poststroke depression. *Journal of Neuropsychiatry & Clinical Neurosciences*, **8**, 399–403.

Murphy, E., Smith, R., Lindesay, J., and Slattery, J. (1988). Increased mortality rates in late-life depression. *British Journal of Psychiatry*, **152**, 347–353.

Musselman, D.L., Evans, D.L., and Nemeroff, C.B. (1998). The relationship of depression to cardiovascular disease: epidemiology, biology, and treatment. *Archives of General Psychiatry*, **55**, 580–592.

Musselman, D.L., Tomer, A., Manatunga, A.K., *et al.* (1996). Exaggerated platelet reactivity in major depression. *American Journal of Psychiatry*, **153**, 1313–1317.

O'Brien, J., Ames, D., Chiu, E., Schweitzer, I., Desmond, P., and Tress, B. (1998). Severe deep white matter lesions and outcome in elderly patients with major depressive disorder: follow up study. *BMJ*, **317**, 982–984.

O'Brien, J., Ames, D., and Schweitzer, I. (1993). HPA axis function in depression and dementia: a review. *International Journal of Geriatric Psychiatry*, **8**, 887–898.

O'Brien, J., Desmond, P., Ames, D., Schweitzer, I., Harrigan, S., and Tress, B. (1996a). A magnetic resonance imaging study of white matter lesions in depression and Alzheimer's disease. *British Journal of Psychiatry*, **168**, 477–485.

O'Brien, J.T., Ames, D., Schweitzer, I., Colman, P., Desmond, P., and Tress, B. (1996b). Clinical and magnetic resonance imaging correlates of hypothalamic-pituitary-adrenal axis function in depression and Alzheimer's disease. *British Journal of Psychiatry*, **168**, 679–687.

Park, S.B., Coull, J.T., McShane, R.H., *et al.* (1994). Tryptophan depletion in normal volunteers produces selective impairments in learning and memory. *Neuropharmacology*, **33**, 575–588.

Paterniti, S., Verdier-Taillefer, M.H., Geneste, C., Bisserbe, J.C., and Alperovitch, A. (2000). Low blood pressure and risk of depression in the elderly. A prospective community-based study. *British Journal of Psychiatry*, **176**, 464–467.

Penninx, B.W., Beekman, A.T., Honig, A., *et al.* (2001). Depression and cardiac mortality: results from a community-based longitudinal study. *Archives of General Psychiatry*, **58**, 221–227.

Penninx, B.W., Geerlings, S.W., Deeg, D.J., van Eijk, J.T., van Tilburg, W., and Beekman, A.T. (1999). Minor and major depression and the risk of death in older persons. *Archives of General Psychiatry*, **56**, 889–895.

Pohjasvaara, T., Leppavuori, A., Siira, I., Vataja, R., Kaste, M., and Erkinjuntti, T. (1998). Frequency and clinical determinants of poststroke depression. *Stroke*, **29**, 2311–2317.

Porter, R.J., Lunn, B.S., Walker, L.L., Gray, J.M., Ballard, C.G., and O'Brien, J.T. (2000). Cognitive deficit induced by acute tryptophan depletion in patients with Alzheimer's disease. *American Journal of Psychiatry*, **157**, 638–640.

Pratt, L.A., Ford, D.E., Crum, R.M., Armenian, H.K., Gallo, J.J., and Eaton, W.W. (1996). Depression, psychotropic medication, and risk of myocardial infarction. Prospective data from the Baltimore ECA follow-up. *Circulation*, **94**, 3123–3129.

Prince, M.J., Harwood, R.H., Blizard, R.A., Thomas, A., and Mann, A.H. (1997a). Impairment, disability and handicap as risk factors for depression in old age. The Gospel Oak Project V. *Psychological Medicine*, **27**, 311–321.

Prince, M.J., Harwood, R.H., Blizard, R.A., Thomas, A., and Mann, A.H. (1997b). Social support deficits, loneliness and life events as risk factors for depression in old age. The Gospel Oak Project VI. *Psychological Medicine*, **27**, 323–332.

Prince, M.J., Harwood, R.H., Thomas, A., and Mann, A.H. (1998). A prospective population-based cohort study of the effects of disablement and social milieu on the onset and maintenance of late-life depression. The Gospel Oak Project VII. *Psychological Medicine*, **28**, 337–350.

Pulska, T., Pahkala, K., Laippala, P., and Kivela, S.L. (1999). Follow up study of longstanding depression as predictor of mortality in elderly people living in the community. *Bmj*, **318**, 432–433.

Rabkin, J.G., Charles, E., and Kass, F. (1983). Hypertension and DSM-III depression in psychiatric outpatients. *American Journal of Psychiatry*, **140**, 1072–1074.

Reding, M., Haycox, J., and Blass, J. (1985). Depression in patients referred to a dementia clinic. A three-year prospective study. *Archives of Neurology*, **42**, 894–896.

Reynolds, C.F., III, Frank, E., Dew, M.A., *et al.* (1999a). Treatment of 70(+)-year-olds with recurrent major depression. Excellent short-term but brittle long-term response. *American Journal of Geriatric Psychiatry*, **7**, 64–69.

Reynolds, C.F., Frank, E., Kupfer, D.J., *et al.* (1996). Treatment outcome in recurrent major depression: a post hoc comparison of elderly ('young old') and midlife patients. *American Journal of Psychiatry*, **153**, 1288–1292.

Reynolds, C.F., III, Frank, E., Perel, J.M., *et al.* (1999*b*). Nortriptyline and interpersonal psychotherapy as maintenance therapies for recurrent major depression: a randomized controlled trial in patients older than 59 years [see comments]. *Jama*, **281**, 39–45.

Roberts, R.E., Kaplan, G.A., Shema, S.J., and Strawbridge, W.J. (1997). Does growing old increase the risk for depression? *American Journal of Psychiatry*, **154**, 1384–1390.

Robinson, R.G., Starr, L.B., Kubos, K.L., and Price, T.R. (1983). A two-year longitudinal study of post-stroke mood disorders: findings during the initial evaluation. *Stroke*, **14**, 736–741.

Robinson, R.G., Starr, L.B., Lipsey, J.R., Rao, K., and Price, T.R. (1985), A two-year longitudinal study of poststroke mood disorders. *Journal of Nervous and Mental Diseases*, **173**, 221–226.

Salloway, S., Malloy, P., Kohn, R., *et al.* (1996). MRI and neuropsychological differences in early- and late-life-onset geriatric depression. *Neurology*, **46**, 1567–1574.

Sapolsky, R.M. (2000). Glucocorticoids and hippocampal atrophy in neuropsychiatric disorders. *Archives of General Psychiatry*, **57**, 925–935.

Sapolsky, R.M., Krey, L.C., and McEwen, B.S. (1986). The neuroendocrinology of stress and aging: the glucocorticoid cascade hypothesis. *Endocrine Reviews*, **7**, 284–301.

Sapolsky, R.M. and Plotsky, P.M. (1990). Hypercortisolism and its possible neural bases. *Biological Psychiatry*, **27**, 937–952.

Sauer, W.H., Mandani, M.M., Wells, P.S., and Williams, S.E. (2001). Selective serotonin reuptake inhibitors and myocardial infarction. *Circulation*, **104**, 1894–1898.

Schoevers, R.A., Beekman, A.T., Deeg, D.J., Geerlings, M.I., Jonker, C., and Van Tilburg, W. (2000*a*). Risk factors for depression in later life; results of a prospective community based study (AMSTEL). *Journal of Affective Disorders*, **59**, 127–137.

Schoevers, R.A., Geerlings, M.I., Beekman, A.T., *et al.* (2000*b*). Association of depression and gender with mortality in old age. Results from the Amsterdam Study of the Elderly (AMSTEL). *British Journal of Psychiatry*, **177**, 336–342.

Schulz, R., Beach, S.R., Ives, D.G., Martire, L.M., Ariyo, A.A., and Kop, W.J. (2000). Association between depression and mortality in older adults: the Cardiovascular Health Study. *Archives of Internal Medicine*, **160**, 1761–1768.

Sharma, V.K., Copeland, J.R., Dewey, M.E., Lowe, D., and Davidson, I. (1998). Outcome of the depressed elderly living in the community in Liverpool: a 5-year follow-up. *Psychological Medicine*, **28**, 1329–1337.

Sheline, Y.I., Sanghavi, M., Mintun, M.A., and Gado, M.H. (1999). Depression duration but not age predicts hippocampal volume loss in medically healthy women with recurrent major depression. *Journal of Neuroscience*, **19**, 5034–5043.

Simonsick, E.M., Wallace, R.B., Blazer, D.G., and Berkman, L.F. (1995). Depressive symptomatology and hypertension-associated morbidity and mortality in older adults. *Psychosomatic Medicine*, **57**, 427–435.

Simpson, S., Baldwin, R.C., Jackson, A., and Burns, A.S. (1998). Is subcortical disease associated with a poor response to antidepressants? Neurological, neuropsychological and neuroradiological findings in late-life depression. *Psychological Medicine*, **28**, 1015–1026.

Simpson, S.W., Jackson, A., Baldwin, R.C., and Burns, A. (1997). 1997 IPA/Bayer research awards in psychogeriatrics. Subcortical hyperintensities in late-life depression: acute response to treatment and neuropsychological impairment. *International Psychogeriatrics*, **9**, 257–275.

Starkman, M.N., Gebarski, S.S., Berent, S., and Schteingart, D.E. (1992). Hippocampal formation volume, memory dysfunction, and cortisol Levels in Patients with Cushing's Syndrome. *Biological Psychiatry*, **32**, 756–765.

Starkman, M.N., Giordani, B., Gebarski, S.S., Berent, S., Schork, M.A., and Schteingart, D.E. (1999). Decrease in cortisol reverses human hippocampal atrophy following treatment of Cushing's disease. *Biological Psychiatry*, **46**, 1595–1602.

Steffens, D.C., Helms, M.J., Krishnan, K.R., and Burke, G.L. (1999). Cerebrovascular disease and depression symptoms in the cardiovascular health study. *Stroke*, **30**, 2159–2166.

Tew, J.D., Jr., Mulsant, B.H., Haskett, R.F., *et al.* (1999). Acute efficacy of ECT in the treatment of major depression in the old-old. *American Journal of Psychiatry*, **156**, 1865–1870.

Thomas, A.J., Ferrier, I.N., Kalaria, R.N., Perry, R.H., Brown, A., and O'Brien, J.T. (2001). A neuropathological study of vascular factors in late-life depression. *Journal of Neurology, Neurosurgery & Psychiatry*, **70**, 83–87.

Thomas, A.J., Ferrier, I.N., Kalaria, R.N., *et al.* (2000). Elevation in late-life depression of intercellular adhesion molecule-1 expression in the dorsolateral prefrontal cortex. *American Journal of Psychiatry*, **157**, 1682–1684.

Thomas, A.J., O'Brien, J.T., and Davis, S., *et al.* (2002). Ischemic basis for deep white matter hyperintensities in major Depression: A Neuropathological Study. *Archives of General Psychiatry* (in press).

Troxler, R.G., Sprague, E.A., Albanese, R.A., Fuchs, R., and Thompson, A.J. (1977). The association of elevated plasma cortisol and early atherosclerosis as demonstrated by coronary angiography. *Atherosclerosis*, **26**, 151–162.

Tutus, A., Simsek, A., Sofuoglu, S., *et al.* (1998). Changes in regional cerebral blood flow demonstrated by single photon emission computed tomography in depressive disorders: comparison of unipolar vs. bipolar subtypes. *Psychiatry Research*, **83**, 169–177.

Uno, H., Tarara, R., Else, J.G., Suleman, M.A., and Sapolsky, R.M. (1989). Hippocampal damage associated with prolonged and fatal stress in primates. *Journal of Neuroscience*, 9, 1705–1711.

Wardle, J., Armitage, J., Collins, R., Wallendszus, K., Keech, A., and Lawson, A. (1996). Randomised placebo controlled trial of effect on mood of lowering cholesterol concentration. Oxford Cholesterol Study Group. *Bmj*, 313, 75–78.

Wassertheil-Smoller, S., Applegate, W.B., Berge, K., *et al.* (1996). Change in depression as a precursor of cardiovascular events. SHEP Cooperative Research Group (Systolic Hypertension in the elderly). *Archives of Internal Medicine*, 156, 553–561.

Weeke, A., Juel, K., and Vaeth, M. (1987). Cardiovascular death and manic-depressive psychosis. *Journal of Affective Disorders*, 13, 287–292.

Wells, C.E. (1979). Pseudodementia. American Journal of *Psychiatry*, 136, 895–900.

Wilson, K., Mottram, P., Sivanranthan, A., and Nightingale, A. (2001). *Cochrane Database of Systematic Reviews*, 2.

Chapter 8

Unipolar depression across the lifespan: issues and prospects

Ian M. Goodyer

The genetics of depression

Over the past two decades behavioural genetic studies involving twins, adoption, and family designs have established a significant genetic contribution to aetiology of the depressions and other complex psychiatric phenotypes (Corsico and McGuffin, 2001). Undertaking genome wide searches as well as determining the strength of associations between susceptibility genes and clinical phenotypes will considerably improve the likelihood of determining the functional genes of interest. In addition the use of quantitative trait markers (QTL) of behaviour that are themselves associated with disorder, will enhance the opportunity for establishing links between molecules, psychology, and psychiatric disorder (Plomin *et al.*, 2001). QTL approaches may delineate the genetically mediated processes that confer liability for clinical impairment. Examples of candidate traits include measures of social cognition in children and adolescents a set of highly heritable traits including the ability to read social situations, and the degree to which understanding and appreciating other peoples perspectives may be genetically influenced (Scourfield *et al.*, 1999). Absence or deficits in such skills is associated with an increased risk for most psychopathologies. A second example is that of a negative emotional temperament which is highly heritable (Eley and Plomin, 1997) and associated with the onset of major depression in adolescents (Goodyer *et al.*, 1993). These studies indicate the possibility that one pathway through which genes may exert their influence is via a set of affective-cognitive processes that are themselves carrying particular risks for subsequent affective disorders. To date investigation applying behavioural genetic methods using sensation seeking and dysfunctional attitudes as the candidate 'psychological hazards' has proven disappointing with little evidence for genetic influences on their association with depression (Farmer et al., 2001a,b). Using psychological traits with high levels of heritability and robust psychometric properties at the level of measurement is likely to considerably improve the success of this promising strategy.

A second potential set of genetic effects are those which increase the liability for environments that provoke psychopathology (Kendler et al., 1995; Kendler and Karkowski-Shuman, 1997). For example, there are clear-cut genetic influences on the occurrence of life events at most ages and stages of development although the exact gene-environment mechanisms remain unclear. (Kendler and Karkowski-Shuman, 1997; Silberg et al., 1999). Kendler and colleagues showed that genetic liability to major unipolar depression in women was associated with a significantly increased risk for six personal (assault, serious marital problems, divorce/breakup, job loss, serious illness, and major financial problems) and one network severe life events (trouble getting along with relatives/friends) (Kendler and Karkowski-Shuman, 1997). Silberg and colleagues noted that the greater heritability for depression in pubertal girls, its genetic mediation over time, and the increase in genetic variance for life events may be one possible explanation for the emergence of increased depression among pubertal girls and its persistence through adolescence (Silberg et al., 1999). These findings underpin the value of searching for the intermediate phenotype of depressive disorders, determining their degree of genetic influence and elucidating the precise genes involved. It is crucial to note that social environmental influences on the liability for depression are not all genetic. Indeed many of the major life events and difficulties (perhaps two-thirds of those reported as highly negative to the self) that contribute to the evolving nature of depressive disorders throughout the lifespan are causal and non-genetic in origin (Kendler et al., 1999).

From the developmental perspective there is good evidence to note that genetic influences for unipolar depression and/or depressive symptoms are greater in adolescence compared with childhood (Eley et al., 1998; Silberg et al., 1999; Rice et al., 2002;). These appear to remain robust throughout the next four decades but it is unclear if depressions in later life are as genetic as the preceding four decades. There is therefore a suggestive inverted U-shaped curve that may best describe genetic liability for depressive disorders over the life-course with the greater effects probably being displayed by disorders beginning after 14 but before 60 years of age, with a strong familial history, recurrent course, high levels of comorbid non-depressive disorders, and functional impairment. Such characteristics do appear to distinguish between subtypes of depression, at least in adult females (Kendler *et al.*, 1994; Kendler *et al.*, 1996).

To date molecular genetic studies have had little success in detecting susceptibility genes for unipolar depressions but some important clues have been elucidated. For example, there is considerable interest in determining the association and functional behavioural effects of the serotonin transporter gene, which is expressed in brain and blood cells, is the site of action of SSRIs and has been the target of a large number of studies since the description of a functional polymorphism in the promoter region. Such a potentially important molecular target remains a site of intense interest for therapeutic advances as well as determining its association with, clinical symptoms, quantitative traits, such as negative temperament, and more directly with aspects of mood and negative cognitions (Lesch, 2001). The serotonin gene contains two allelic variants a long (ll) and a short form giving three known possible combinations ll, ls, and ss. A significant association has been reported between the l homozygous genotype and the depressive response to TRP depletion (Moreno *et al.*, 2002). Individuals whose genotype predicted increased 5-HT transporter activity may be more susceptible to depressive changes in response to transient 5-HT perturbations. There is currently uncertainty on the precise allelic variations of the serotonin transporter gene that are of importance as the s-allele (both homo- and heterozygous forms) together with a positive family history of major unipolar depression have also been shown to act as additive risk factors for the depressive response following tryptophan depletion (Neumeister *et al.*, 2002). The findings demonstrate the potential for clarifying the relation between genetic risk for depression and a physiological challenge test. The use of genotyping for challenge tests may reduce the non-response to tryptophan depletion by selecting a more homogeneous subset of participants. Whether such an approach will predict greater response to antidepressants and therefore inform therapeutic choice and clinical management remains to be established.

To date it remains unclear which variations in the serotonin transporter system contribute to the liability for the onset of depression. As yet no prospective studies have reported the potential additive effects of allelic variation in the presence of other known environmental risk factors for subsequent affective psychopathology. From Chapters 2 and 3 in this volume one might predict that the preliminary findings regarding the association between the ll form of the serotonin transporter would be replicated in adolescent but perhaps less so in child depression which appears to be biologically somewhat different from similar depressive phenotypes at different stages in the lifespan.

Finally there may be opportunities to determine the role of functionally important genes in psychological challenge tests. This may help to elucidate the intermediate psychology in subjects at risk for disorder or, as with the tryptophan depletion test, improve the specificity of experimental studies looking for genetic traits underpinning response to mood induction or other stimulus paradigms used to evoke dysphoria and negative cognitions about the self. Incorporating genotyping into challenge studies and looking for associations within families and sib-pairs as well as differences between case and controls or high and low risk subjects is clearly an important strategy that should be included in many studies in the near future. The use of such genotyping in prospective community studies would seem highly desirable.

Such studies in the future are unlikely to be confined to the serotonin transporter. Monoamine genes in general clearly require serious consideration as targets for the common psychopathologies involving affect dysfunction. For example, a functional polymorphism, the long allelic form of MAO-A, has recently been found to be associated with unipolar depression in females suggesting elevated MAO-A activity for some individuals with major depressive disorder (Schulze *et al.*, 2000). Equally there may be different genetic constituents operating differentially across the lifespan in part perhaps as a component of the ageing process. For example, in a recent study of late onset depressions (median age 55 years) there was an increased rate of the C677T mutation of the methylenetetrahydrofolate reductase enzyme (MTHFR) gene mutation together with vascular risk factors. This suggests that a proportion of these patients, having perhaps their first unipolar episode in some cases, may have a disorder that is part related to different genes than those of similar disorders occurring in earlier life. Perhaps genes influencing the liability to vascular disease are themselves more relevant to disorders in late life. Finally it is important to remember that basic molecular genetics and genomics in human biology continue to gather new knowledge at an enormous rate. Whether the clinical genetic studies to date have truly been able to target the important functional polymorphisms of interest, or even the right genes, remains to be firmly established. This is already one of the most exciting and important areas for depression research across the lifespan and with greater collaboration with basic molecular genetics is likely to yield crucial information regarding the nature of affective disorders.

The formation of risk

Social origins of depression

Over the past three decades there has been a focus on the environmental origins of depression. Perhaps the most influential studies were those of Brown and Harris (Brown and Harris, 1978) who introduced extensive psychosocial interviewing procedures with epidemiological approaches to ascertain women at risk for and/or suffering with major depression. There was already an important literature pointing to the fact that life events with a high negative effect on the individual and occurring in the months prior to a clinically definable onset of depression were important precipitants of disorder (Paykel *et al.*, 1969; Paykel, 1978). Brown and Harris extended these findings proposing that there was a definable psychological a construct, that of personal threat, embedded within the social context of a negative life experience that was specifically associated with the onset of major depression. Importantly they showed that only a proportion of women, those with pre-existing serious chronic social adversities exposed to such highly threatening life events and difficulties were truly 'at risk' for the onset of major depression. Various refinements have subsequently taken place but the necessary social model is one of a vulnerable individual whose social environment is predisposing them to a high risk for the onset of depression but which can only be brought about by a proximally occurring highly negative personal experience that is unexpected and threatens the already low level of well-being to provoke the onset of major depression.

As already noted one critical refinement from behavioural genetic studies is that individuals may, through their own behaviours, bring about negative life events on themselves (Kendler and Karkowski-Shuman, 1997). These person-dependent events need to be considered theoretically differently from negative events that occur independently of self-behaviour. A second inference from genetic studies is that the sensitivity of an individual to events is itself genetically mediated (Kendler *et al.*, 1995). This implies that there will be marked individual differences in response to the same form and intensity of negative life events. Whilst these refinements are important the basic social model proposed by Brown and originally intimated by Paykel and colleagues (Paykel *et al.*, 1969) is quite robust (Fergusson and Horwood, 1987). The model appears to be relatively applicable across the lifespan although around half of first episode major depressions in adolescence arise from chronic psychosocial adversities without clear-cut exposure to provoking event (Goodyer *et al.*, 2000). This suggests that first episode unipolar depressions have a somewhat different set of environmental formation processes to account for both slow growing and fast onset disorders with the same broad clinical phenotype (Rueter *et al.*, 1999; Goodyer, 2002).

Parent–child interactions

Over the past ten years it has become increasingly apparent that the early years of postnatal life are setting up some individuals for evoking their own negative life events in the second and third decades of life. Murray and Cooper (Chapter 2 this volume) outline how the intergenerational transmission of psychological characteristics from parent to infant and young child could bring some of these hazards about. These authors highlighted the importance of persisting positive affiliative ties in the formation of socially competent children to reduce negative self-percept by middle childhood. Whilst the psychological mechanisms require further elucidation it appears that the formation of competence involves the child evolving two efficient sets of psychological processing, social sensitivity, and performance functions. The notion is that mental coherence arises developmentally from the interplay between evolving social cognition and cognitive control processes leading to the child being ably to select a competent behavioural strategy at times of social challenge or demand. It is important to note that the child is an active participant in this process and indeed from the first few weeks of life will have innate genetically mediated abilities that are 'hard wired' to dissect maternal or paternal cues some of which will be confusing and unpredictable. It appears that early environmental risks for subsequent emotion psychopathologies involve a failure to organize infant behaviour that is required to facilitate interpersonal relations. The hypothesis is that this occurs because of poorly formed mental coherence between social sensitivity and performance functions whose evolving nature depends on early parental cues and interactions. The evidence for the importance of mental coherence is emerging from developmental studies.

Clearly genetically mediated behavioural styles in the infant can moderate the effects of parental behaviour. Difficult infant temperament is associated with high rates of psychopathology over the childhood years. During adolescence and throughout the next four decades of adult life high levels of emotionality (consists of: easily brought to tears, often makes a fuss, easily upset, reacting intensely when upset, tends to be emotional) and/or neuroticism are associated with an increased risk for affective disorders although there is no exact specificity of that intrinsic risk to the form of emotional disorder (Hirshfeld et al., 1992; Goodyer et al., 1993; Caspi et al., 1995, 1997). Murray and Cooper also remind us that early parent–infant processes are crucial mediating experiences in the evolving nature of temperament and that some of the important regulating processes, such as the development of attention and working memory arise in the child through regulatory processes emanating from the caretaker. There has been little investigation of the evolving development of these executive processes in the first two decades of life although general memory functions and perhaps some attentional processing components such as searching and selection reach adult type levels by eight years of age (Gathercole, 1998; Luciana and Nelson, 1998; Nelson, 1998). From the psychopathological perspective the role of dysregulations within the psychological systems of memory, behavioural inhibition and decision making in the development of unipolar depression remains unclear. By contrast their putative importance in adult depression has become a focus of considerable interest at least as a concomitant and consequence of unipolar depressive disorders (Murphy *et al.*, 1998; Austin *et al.*, 2001*a*).

It is also apparent that for a proportion of children exposed to parenting difficulties social demands that involve challenge and potential disappointment (as shown in the 'snap' card game paradigm, Murray *et al.*, 2001) can reveal a weak or negative self-percept in which the 'threat' of failure is easily perceived and associated with increasing dysphoric mood.

Thus there is a clear potential pathway for risk in the formative years for two critical psychological processing models of the environment to be developmentally compromised, social sensitivity processes and cognitive performance. If the genetically mediated aspects of behavioural style are important in this regard then those most at risk for these processes will be children with high levels of emotionality in their temperament. Much greater clarification is required regarding the links between temperamental traits and the evolving nature of cognitive skills, such as behavioural inhibition or decision-making and information processing of the social environment.

The implication is that it is these temperamentally at risk children who will go into young adult development carrying the psychological liability to increase, through their own behaviours, the social adversities that form the environmental framework for subsequent onsets of major depression. But whether it is possible to predict that all such children remain at risk for person-dependent life events that lead specifically to depressive disorders is not known.

Thresholder changes

Very little is known in general about the normative transitional processes between late adolescence and early adulthood. Crossing the threshold into adult life has become increasingly complex and the period between school-leaving and independent living (18–25 years) may hold turning points, good and bad, as young adults try to make more permanent decisions about their personal and work lives, and set about disengaging from their parents without necessarily breaking close affiliative ties. The importance of some of these issues for unipolar depression in early adult life were discussed by Lewinsohn and Seeley in Chapter 4 using data from their longitudinal cohort study, the Oregon Depression Project.

These authors noted the critical importance of interpersonal disappointments in subjects who place an emotional reliance in others in the onset of depression in late adolescence and young adults. The personality issues involved in this process remain somewhat unclear but the longitudinal findings show clearly that there continues to be formation of more internal psychological risk processes as young onset depressives and those at risk for affective disorders, move into early adult life. These longitudinal data across the transition from adolescence to early adulthood also demonstrate the negative effects of unipolar depression on adult functioning for both sexes, as those with previous affective disorder histories have smaller social networks and poorer physical health increasing the liability for 'adult' social vulnerabilities described as critical components for episodes of depression in women (Brown *et al.*, 1987).

HPA axis activity over the lifespan

Depressive disorders at most ages show abnormalities in the regulation of hypothalamic-pituitary-adrenal activity. Cortisol hypersecretion, with concomitant loss of the regulatory feedback mechanisms, also appear to show a developmental lifespan trend being more common in the ageing than the younger brain (Lupien *et al.*, 1998; Lupien *et al.*, 1999). This may explain the increased liability for such findings in later life depression discussed in Chapter 7 in this volume. HPA axis abnormalities of a similar characteristic (high levels of evening cortisol secretion) do occur in younger depressions as well (see Chapters 2 and 3). The extent to which the natural developmental liability for inefficient HPA axis function occurs with age may be influenced by the risk processes that promote the onset of unipolar depressions. Thus the origins of these HPA axis difficulties during an episode of disorder may in some cases arise in individuals with high levels of social adversity in earlier life resulting in a more labile corticoid response system. For example, some young individuals may be exposed to qualitatively highly difficult and stressful early circumstances that compromise neural development (Gunnar, 1998). Thus early life events may influence subsequent cortisol reactivity in man, as in experimental animals (Vazquez, 1998). In the latter, early adverse events such as separation from the mother can have long-lasting effects on glucocorticoid reactivity in adult life (Anisman *et al.*, 1998). Alternatively as already noted, there may be a direct effect of ageing on regulatory mechanisms making this hormone dysregulation more likely with age. A third possibility is that major depression itself, if untreated or running a chronic relapsing course exerts deleterious effects on brain function as evinced by poor control of cortisol dynamics at subsequent episodes. Currently it is unclear if any or all of these mechanisms contribute to depressions at different ages and stages of development.

Corticoid-cognitive dysfunction

Cortisol hypersecretion is clearly not a trivial issue as functional and structural impairments to the brain and to the hippocampus in particular, arise as a consequence of exposure to chronically high cortisol levels and these are likely to have relevance for affective-cognitive impairments in man (Sapolsky, 2000; Roozendaal *et al.*, 2001; Patel *et al.*, 2002). The most frequently reported corticoid-related cognitive impairment in humans to date are those involving impairments in declarative memory functions (Lupien *et al.*, 1998; Newcomer *et al.*, 1999). The ageing brain may be more susceptible to such corticoid effects in part because of the potential decline in neuroprotection that may occur in the central nervous system over time (Guazzo *et al.*, 1996; Lupien *et al.*, 1998; Kimonides *et al.*, 1999). In such circumstances relatively less negative events (social risks, infections, illnesses, drug induced, etc.) will be required to initiate abnormalities in interpersonal social cognition, such as lower empathy and less ability to appreciate the perspective of others, or in mental performance such as episodic memory, problem solving, and behavioural inhibition. Thus it seems probable that, at the psychological level of risk, corticoid-related memory impairments occur at all ages but are in part developmentally mediated with greater sensitivity for such seen in the elderly. High circulating cortisol levels are already known to contribute to the onset and pathophysiology of first episode unipolar depressions (Harris *et al.*, 2000; Goodyer *et al.*, 2001). It is not known if corticoid-memory interactions arise in well individuals that may predispose them to subsequent first episode or recurrent unipolar disorders.

Depression induced neural sensitivity

A second notion is that risk processes require fewer socially adverse precipitants with increasingly recurrent episodes because of the neural effects arising from the first episode. This may be explained by the hypothesis that cortisol hypersecretion is itself a risk for recurrence through alterations in the biochemical and anatomical substrates underlying the affective disorders (Post, 1992). Thus HPA axis impairments may evolve over time in the younger subjects as a function of recurrences. The subpopulation at risk for recurrent unipolar depressions in later life may therefore be those with a greater neurotoxic response to cortisol via two additive processes, ageing and the effects of recurrent depression on HPA axis sensitivity. Whether there is a true-dose response type curve over time that suggests less social adversity is required to produce clinical depression is not entirely clear. Furthermore as noted by Paykel and Kennedy in Chapter 6, individuals in mid and late life are undoubtedly exposed to many adversities and many unipolar disorders in midlife are first episodes, suggesting there may be some specific qualities regarding the nature of life events in these age ranges that are important in the genesis of an episode of unipolar depression.

In addition however these authors noted that the less common psychotic forms of unipolar depression appear to be more frequent from midlife and may arise without the same overt levels of social adversity either proximally or distally from earlier years. This suggests that there may be different mechanisms involved in the onset of these severe forms of unipolar depressions that are influenced by a change in risks occurring from the third decade of life onwards. As well as psychotic features, the characteristics of more common depressions may alter with age, for example, with greater emphasis on physical symptoms as suggested from studies in the elderly (Chapter 7). Thus many episodes of psychotic or severe depressions with high levels of physical symptoms, occur in adults with prior psychiatric histories and compromised neuro-cognitive functions. There are others that may be more *de novo* whose aetiology remains more obscure.

Mental dysfunctions and depression

The search for clear-cut patterns of mental impairments that predict the onset of unipolar depression is another area of intense research in depression (Teasdale and Barnard, 1993; Murphy *et al.*, 1998; Teasdale *et al.*, 1998). The development of tasks that are available for use in functional neuroimaging studies to determine the precise neural correlates that underpin both aetiological and pathophysiological processes is beginning to delineate the neural pathways that are likely to be involved (Drevets, 2001; Elliott *et al.*, 2002). It is increasingly apparent that coherence of brain systems involved in the recognition, processing, and response formation to emotionally meaningful stimuli from the environment is required to prevent inefficient mental functions. Exactly how these neural systems operate to process affectively valent information is slowly emerging but we remain relatively ignorant of the precise psychological processes that if not functioning will result in depressive disorders. It seems highly likely that fully integrated social and performance functions are needed and that a breakdown in one or more component involved in processing environmental stimuli may result in unipolar major depression perhaps through a failure to adequately process incoming environmental stimuli (Goodyer, 2002).

Memory and depression

Biases in episodic event memory processes are one obvious aspect of information processing likely to mediate the liability for subsequent psychopathology. Episodic memory includes context rich memories relating to the self, known as 'autobiographical' memory whose neural basis is closely associated with the hippocampus (Mishkin et al., 1997). There is evidence that in depressed adults, deficits in episodic (autobiographical) memory processes relate to poor social problem solving (Evans et al., 1992). Deficits in autobiographical memory retrieval predict persistence of major depressive disorder, (Brittlebank et al., 1993). The ontogeny of these types of memories are not known, although autobiographical memories may arise during infancy (Harley and Reese, 1999) with adult-type memory function present by the age of eight (Gathercole, 1998). Early adverse experiences, such as child maltreatment or maternal deprivation, may have undesirable consequences for memory development (Lynch and Cicchetti, 1998; Pollak et al., 1998), but whether these events operate through effects on brain as a consequence of changes in adrenal steroid function is unclear.

The nature of memory impairment, and executive function deficits, may depend on the form of disorder as compared with milder and more common depressive disorders severe melancholic adult depressives show a more widespread pattern of impairments including working memory and selective attention (Austin et al.1999; Austin et al., 2001b). Overall there does seem to be considerable evidence that memory deficitis and/or distortions of social experience contributing to the nature of unipolar depressions at most ages but the nature and characteristics of these and their specificity to unipolar depressions at different ages remains unclear. For example, autobiographical deficits in episodic memory have been noted in first episode depressions during adolescence but the associations are not straightforward being positively correlated with the severity of the episode and general intelligence but no more likely in depression than in patients with current non affective psychiatric syndromes (Park et al., 2002).

Whether these deficits precede the onset of major depressions and do so systematically at different stages in the lifespan is not known. In addition it is not clear what the relational pattern of performance difficulties are within existing unipolar depressions. Thus the observation that there are widespread executive dysfunctions in current depressive disorders is important (Murphy et al., 1998) but cannot inform us if, for example, episodic memory difficulties will only become problematic in individuals with preceding selective attentional dysfunctions with the resultant failure to remove unwanted and harmful thoughts about the self from consciousness.

With respect to depression what we need to determine specifically are the molecular and neural mechanisms that result in (a) selective bias of negative information processing about the self, (b) how this is activated in some individuals following mild dysphoria, and (c) what is deficient such that these depressogenic process cannot be 'switched off'. Longitudinal studies of subjects at high risk for major depression followed through the evolving nature of the disorder to either recovery or remission would be able to elucidate the sequential nature and characteristics of the pathological psychological processes.

Emotion and depression

Emotion recognition and response elements are also likely to be important in the aetiology and pathophysiology of depressions. Whilst emotion psychology has only recently found itself back in favour in the clinical neurosciences it is increasingly apparent that the amygdala has a critical role in the recognition of basic emotions such as fear, disgust, and probably sadness and that deficits in function are likely to compromise normal emotion processing (Calder *et al.*, 2001). Increased blood flow and glucose metabolism in the left amygdala is positively correlated with cortisol levels in subjects with familial depressions reflecting either the effect of amygdala activity on corticotropin-releasing hormone (CRH) secretion or the effect of cortisol on amygdala function (Drevets *et al.*, 2002). Moderate doses (but not high ones) of glucocorticoids also enhance the consolidation of memory for emotionally charged experiences (McEwen and Sapolsky, 1995). This effect depends on the amygdala, and is prevented by blocking their actions within this structure. The amygdala, in turn, is closely associated with other parts of the brain known to be implicated in emotion, such as the orbital part of the frontal lobe (McDonald, 1998; McDonald *et al.*, 1999).

Neurocognitive systems, cortisol, and depression

In early-onset major depression brain changes have been reported in the hippocampus, amygdala, caudate nucleus, putamen, and frontal cortex structures (the limbic-cortical-striatal-pallidal-thalamic tract -LSCPT) (Drevets, 1999) (Mayberg *et al.*, 1999; Liotti *et al.*, 2000) (Bremner *et al.*, 2000). Of these structures, volume loss in the hippocampus is the only consistently observed change to persist past the resolution of the depression (Sheline, 2000). Possible mechanisms for tissue loss include exposure to repeated episodes of hypercortisolemia. Increases in amygdala metabolism and a positive correlation with peripheral cortisol levels during major depression has been noted indicating that this too may be a glucocorticoid sensitive brain area (Drevets, 1999). FMRI with healthy volunteers and patients has shown that the amygdala is particularly involved in processing facial expressions of fear (Morris *et al.*, 1996; Phillips *et al.*, 1997; Whalen *et al.*, 1998; Calder *et al.*, 2001). Significant decreases in the amygdala signal are also produced by viewing happy facial expressions (Morris *et al.*, 1996, 1998; Whalen *et al.*, 1998). In procaine-induced emotions fear is *positively* and euphoria *negatively* correlated with left amygdala rCBF (Ketter *et al.*, 1996). The amygdala is also involved with the formation of enhanced declarative memory for emotionally arousing events that are contextually processed via the hippocampus (Cahill and McGaugh, 1998). Thus the amygdala-hippocampal connections of the LSCPT are rich in glucocorticoid receptors (Evans and Arriza, 1989) making them sensitive to abnormal cortisol levels and thereby potentially influencing fear and happiness recognition and episodic memory.

Whether these neural and psychoendocrine links are present in high risk subjects prior to the onset of a major depressive episode is not known. Neither is it clear if the neurocognitive deficits and cortisol abnormalities are likely to occur in all forms of major depression or more likely in those, for example, with a history of past depressive episode with cortisol hypersecretion.

Therapeutics

Public health implications

From the clinical and public health perspective there is certainly hope for the future. Considerable effort and expenditure is already being made in many countries worldwide to improve parenting and infant well-being. Murray and Cooper (Chapter 2) demonstrate that parenting skills are crucial in ameliorating the potential hazards to the infant of post-natal depression and its consequences for parent–child relations. Positive emotional relations between parent and child can be taught but the policy decisions that determine how best this should be carried out remain unresolved. A universal educational approach might involve the teaching of parent skills in schools as part of the general educational curriculum. A similar universal strategy would be to provide parent-craft lessons to all new mothers rather than on a volunteer or first come first served basis. Such lessons would however be psychological in nature as well as focussed on physical and instrumental care. Such universal programmes would be expensive, requiring skilled teachers and therapists, and a plentiful supply of both. Would the benefits outweigh the costs? Perhaps, but there is little evidence at this time and there would be considerable competition for health care funds from many other quarters. There is a need to try and establish through a randomized controlled trial in the community at large if such a universal parenting strategy would improve infant well-being using outcome measures in the child known to be related to subsequent liability for affective disorders.

Such a programme could and should make use of self-help information and education programmes delivered, for example, through interactive CD-Rom procedures. Designing a package that explained child emotional development, how parent–infant processes were important for the right early developmental trajectory and recognizing the signs in both the parents and the infants that might indicate interrelationships were not going well and what to do about that, could be incorporated and evaluated in such a trial. Diminishing the risks for subsequent emotional and behavioural difficulties with an effective universal early parenting programme would be a marked step in the right direction for child mental development in primary health care settings. Without an evidence base for such a strategy, available most effectively through a randomized control trial, it may be harder to persuade governments to promote such a universal policy at the tax payers expense. Targeted programmes, for example, for infants at risk for poor child development in general, are already an accepted part of child health policy world wide. Their effectiveness is unclear with regard to mental development although clearly a well nourished and clothed child who has not been maltreated enters middle childhood and adolescence in a physically competent state and is less likely to show emotional difficulties. Interestingly poor fetal growth is associated with increased lability in cortisol secretion in adult life and an increased risk for hypertension and type-2 diabetes (Phillips et al., 2000; Phillips, 2001). These latter findings could have considerable potential implications for psychopathology and complement the findings of Lewinsohn and Seeley who noted much poorer physical health in their risk factors and correlates of first episode onsets of major depression. It is not clear if poor physical growth in antenatally or in early childhood is a major direct correlate for emotional well-being once psychosocial adversities of known importance have been taken into account. Entering adult life with high cortisol levels as a consequence of poor childhood physical a health deserves a closer investigation than given hitherto. Even if there was a significant additive correlation of small effect, it would be conceivable that such a physical risk process for mental development could be alleviated through adequate nutrition both antenatally and postnatally.

General universal mental health programmes for adults are now a well accepted form of delivering information to the public, charities, support groups, and governments all participate although there are few systematically delivered programmes aimed at reducing the risk for unipolar depression in the population at large. It is likely that these will improve and continue to deliver informed information to the public about reducing risks for depression, where to seek help and what to do if one is depressed.

Psychological treatments

For the depressed individual it is apparent that there are now effective psychological treatments. It seems that in the pre-pubertal child these may be more effective than current pharmacological agents which appear markedly less therapeutic in this age range than at any other. O'Brien in Chapter 7 noted that psychological treatments may be underused in later life depressions perhaps because mental health professionals may believe, incorrectly, that older persons are not cognitively able to tolerate treatments like CBT. In fact it appears that treatment response may be better that professionals are aware of and since many older patients may not tolerate medication psychological treatments should perhaps be considered earlier than they often are. As O'Brien points out depression is associated with considerable morbidity and mortality in later life and effective psychological treatments may result in preventable premature deaths. Greater interest in psychological treatments across the lifespan should be encouraged as a component of a comprehensive protocol for treating an episode of depression and in relapse prevention and long term management.

Pharmacological treatments

Between the second and the seventh decade there is increasing evidence for the effectiveness of antidepressant medication. Efficacy may be somewhat positively correlated with age. There are clearly patients who respond less well than others to serotonin re-uptake inhibitors with treatment effects appearing minimal. Paykel and Kennedy's excellent summary (Chapter 6) of the state of the art of antidepressant treatment in mid life notes that overall the response to antidepressants in patients presenting to mental health services is good but recurrence and relapse rates are high. It is encouraging to note that despite these ongoing problems the suicide rate (at least in midlife) has been declining amongst depressives since the 1940s. Whilst this cannot be attributed specifically to treatment with medication the introduction of antidepressants has clearly had a major positive effect on morbidity and mortality across the lifespan.

A major task for treatment is the prevention of relapse and recurrence at all stages of life. There is considerable promise in more comprehensive treatment protocols that combine antidepressants and some psychological treatments and taking a longer view on the role of active management. Thus recent evidence supports a period of 9 months to 1 year for the maintenance of antidepressants after remission (Paykel, 2001). Antidepressants are also effective in maintenance treatment for recurrent depression, and are indicated where there is clear risk of further episodes

(Paykel, 2001). Paykel has recently suggested that antidepressant withdrawal after continuation and maintenance should always be gradual, over a minimum of 3 months and longer after longer maintenance periods, to avoid withdrawal symptoms or rebound relapse. Trials of interpersonal therapy for the prevention of recurrence show some benefit, but effects are weaker than those of drug and additional benefit in combination is limited. There is better evidence for effects of cognitive behaviour therapy in preventing relapse and an emerging indication for its addition to antidepressants, particularly where residual symptoms are present (Jarrett et al., 2001).

The principles of longer term treatment also appear to apply to the elderly with respect to the prevention of recurrence (Klysner et al., 2002) but it is less clear if the same principles should apply to younger onset depressive disorders. One may speculate however that given the high relapse rate following first episode disorders in adolescence, the impairments discussed by Lewinsohn and Seeley (Chapter 4 this volume) and reported by Fombonne and colleagues in their follow-up of child and adolescent depressions (Fombonne et al., 2001) that similar issues should be considered in young adolescent depressed patients. There is certainly little doubt that first episode disorders in the younger age group are at risk from persistent disorder that does not appear to be responding in all cases to brief multidisciplinary treatments (Goodyer et al., 2001).

What seems less clear is how to determine which patients with depression are at risk for recurrent or relapsing disorder. Clinical signs and symptoms do not appear to be particularly predictive in this regard. Perhaps a greater degree of specificity for treatments selection will come from a more comprehensive understanding of the intermediate biology of these heterogeneous conditions.

Some clues can be found in recent attempts to relate serotonin abnormalities to treatment response although the findings are far from consistent with both positive and negative studies reported (Lotrich et al., 2001; Neumeister et al., 2002). For example, allelic variation in the serotonin transporter gene promoter region polymorphism (5-HTTLPR) may contribute to the variable initial response of elderly depressed patients treated with a selective serotonin reuptake inhibitor (Pollock et al., 2000). The clinical effects of the polymorphisms may be associated with effects on platelets, neural 5-HTT levels, and indices of serotonergic function (Lotrich et al., 2001). There is also increasing evidence that serotonin receptor numbers and functions are age sensitive potentially declining from the second or third decade of life and this may influence response to antidepressants as well as variations in the form and outcome of depression (Meyer et al., 2001; Harrison, 2002; Yamamoto et al., 2002). One can expect considerable advances in the near future regarding our understanding of genetic markers for treatment response. The use of genome wide searches as well as a candidate gene approach, will considerably increase the opportunity for detecting genes of interest for indexing therapeutic response to current treatments as well as promoting the search for new therapies based on a much more complete understanding of the genetics of unipolar depressions. It is likely that a greater understanding of the biological bases of these disorders will also enhance the appropriate use of psychological and social therapies. Differentiating the subtypes of affective disorders may then become increasingly possible in routine clinical practice. Overall there are considerable grounds for optimism in improving the treatment of early onset, recurrent, and resistant unipolar depressions across the lifespan, and reducing the long term morbidity and mortality as associated with these complex psychiatric disorders. Unipolar depressions are a major cause of physical and social burden worldwide and it is to be hoped that comprehensive public health and mental health services, together with support for research into the aetiology nature and outcome of these complex disorders, will receive greater support than hitherto for the improved well-being of generations to come.

Acknowledgement

This chapter was completed whilst the Author was in receipt of a Wellcome Trust Programme Grant and member of the MRC(UK) co-operative in Brain, Behaviour and Neuropsychiatry at the University of Cambridge.

References

Anisman, H., Zaharia, M.D., Meaney, M.J., *et al.* (1998). Do early-life events permanently alter behavioral and hormonal responses to stressors? *International Journal of Developmental Neuroscience*, **16**, 149–164.

Austin, M.-P., Mitchell, P., and Goodwin, G. (2001*a*). Cognitive deficits in depression. *British Journal of Psychiatry*, **178**, 200–206.

Austin, M.P., Mitchell, P., and Goodwin, G.M. (2001*b*). Cognitive deficits in depression: possible implications for functional neuropathology. *British Journal of Psychiatry*, **178**, 200–206.

Austin, M.P., Mitchell, P., Wilhelm, K., *et al.* (1999). Cognitive function in depression: a distinct pattern of frontal impairment in melancholia? *Psychological Medicine*, **29**, 73–85.

Bremner, J.D., Narayan, M., Anderson, E.R., *et al.* (2000). Hippocampal volume reduction in major depression. *American Journal of Psychiatry*, **157**, 115–118.

Brittlebank, A.D., Scott, J., Williams, J.M., *et al.* (1993). Autobiographical memory in depression: state or trait marker? [see comments]. *British Journal of Psychiatry*, **162**, 118–121.

Brown, G.W., Bifulco, A., and Harris, T. (1987). Life events, vulnerability and the onset of depression: some refinements. *British Journal of Psychiatry*, **150**, 30–42.

Brown, G.W. and Harris, T. (1978). *Social Origins of Depression: A Study of Psychiatric Disorder in Women.* Tavistock Publications, London.

Cahill, L. and McGaugh, J.L. (1998). Mechanisms of emotional arousal and lasting declarative memory. *Trends in Neuroscience*, **21**, 294–299.

Calder, A., Lawrence, A.D., and Young, A.W. (2001). Neuropsychology of fear and loathing. *Nature*, **2**, 351–363.

Caspi, A., Begg, D., Dickson, N., et al. (1997). Personality differences predict health-risk behaviors in young adulthood: evidence from a longitudinal study. *Journal of Personality and Social Psychology*, **73**, 1052–1063.

Caspi, A., Henry, B., McGee, R.O., et al. (1995). Temperamental origins of child and adolescent behavior problems: from age three to age fifteen. *Child Development*, **66**, 55–68.

Corsico, A. and McGuffin, P. (2001). Psychiatric genetics: recent advances and clinical implications. *Epidemioligica Psychiatrica*, **10**, 253–259.

Drevets, W.C. (1999). Prefrontal cortical-amygdalar metabolism in major depression. *Annals of New York Academy of Science*, **877**, 614–637.

Drevets, W.C. (2001). Neuroimaging and neuropathological studies of depression: implications for the cognitive-emotional features of mood disorders. *Current Opinion in Neurobiology*, **11**, 240–249.

Drevets, W.C., Price, J.L., Bardgett, M.E., et al. (2002). Glucose metabolism in the amygdala in depression: relationship to diagnostic subtype and plasma cortisol levels. *Pharmacology Biochemistry and Behaviour*, **71**, 431–447.

Eley, T.C., Deater-Deckard, K., Fombonne, E., et al. (1998). An adoption study of depressive symptoms in middle childhood. *Journal of Child Psychology and Psychiatry*, **39**, 337–345.

Eley, T.C. and Plomin, R. (1997). Genetic analyses of emotionality. *Current Opinion in Neurobiology*, **7**, 279–284.

Elliott, R., Rubinsztein, J.S., Sahakian, B.J., et al. (2002). The neural basis of mood-congruent processing biases in depression. *Archives of General Psychiatry*, **59**, 597–604.

Evans, J., Williams, J.M., O'Loughlin, S., et al. (1992). Autobiographical memory and problem-solving strategies of parasuicide patients. *Psychological Medicine*, **22**, 399–405.

Evans, R.M. and Arriza, J.L. (1989). A molecular framework for the actions of glucocorticoid hormones in the nervous system. *Neuron*, **2**, 1105–1112.

Farmer, A., Harris, T., Redman, K., et al. (2001a). The cardiff depression study: a sib-pair study of dysfunctional attitudes in depressed probands and healthy control subjects. *Psychological Medicine*, **31**, 627–633.

Farmer, A., Redman, K., Harris, T., et al. (2001b). Sensation-seeking, life events and depression. The cardiff depression study. *British Journal of Psychiatry*, **178**, 549–552.

Fergusson, D.M. and Horwood, L.J. (1987). Vulnerability to life events exposure. *Psychological Medicine*, **17**, 739–749.

Fombonne, E., Wostear, G., Cooper, V., et al. (2001). The Maudsley long-term follow-up of child and adolescent depression. 1. Psychiatric outcomes in adulthood. *British Journal of Psychiatry*, **179**, 210–217.

Gathercole, S.E. (1998). The development of memory. *Journal of Child Psychology and Psychiatry*, **39**, 3–27.

Goodyer, I.M. (2002). Social adversity and mental functions in adolescents at high risk for psychopathology. *British Journal of Psychiatry*, **181**, 1–4.

Goodyer, I.M., Ashby, L., Altham, P.M.E., et al. (1993). Temperament and major depression in 11–16 year olds. *Journal of Child Psychology and Psychiatry*, **34**, 1409–1423.

Goodyer, I.M., Herbert, J., Tamplin, A., et al. (2000). Recent life events, cortisol, dehydroepiandrosterone and the onset of major depression in high-risk adolescents. *British Journal of Psychiatry*, **177**, 499–504.

Goodyer, I.M., Park, R.J., and Herbert, J. (2001). Psychosocial and endocrine features of chronic first-episode major depression in 8–16 year olds. *Biological Psychiatry*, **50**, 351–357.

Goodyer, I.M., Park, R.J., Netherton, C.M., et al. (2001). Possible role of cortisol and dehydroepiandrosterone in human development and psychopathology. *British Journal of Psychiatry*, **179**, 243–249.

Guazzo, E.P., Kirkpatrick, P.J., Goodyer, I.M., et al. (1996). Cortisol, dehydroepandrosterone (DHEA), and DHEA sulfate in the cerebrospinal fluid of man: relation to blood levels and the effects of age. *Journal of Clinical Endocrinology and Metabolism*, **81**, 3951–3960.

Gunnar, M.R. (1998). Quality of early care and buffering of neuroendocrine stress reactions: potential effects on the developing human brain. *Preventative Medicine*, **27**, 208–211.

Harley, K. and Reese, E. (1999). Origins of autobiographical memory. *Developmental Psychology*, **35**, 1338–1348.

Harris, T.O., Borsanyi, S., Messari, S., et al. (2000). Morning cortisol as a risk factor for subsequent major depressive disorder in adult women. *British Journal of Psychiatry*, **177**, 505–510.

Harrison, P.J. (2002). The neuropathology of primary mood disorder. *Brain*, **125**, 1428–1449.

Hirshfeld, D.R., Rosenbaum, J.F., Biederman, J., et al. (1992). Stable behavioral inhibition and its association with anxiety disorder. *Journal of the American Academy of Child and Adolescent Psychiatry*, **31**, 103–111.

Jarrett, R.B., Kraft, D., Doyle, J., et al. (2001). Preventing recurrent depression using cognitive therapy with and without a continuation phase: a randomized clinical trial. *Archives of General Psychiatry*, **58**, 381–388.

Kendler, K.S., Eaves, L.J., Walters, E.E., et al. (1996). The identification and validation of distinct depressive syndromes in a population-based sample of female twins. *Archives of General Psychiatry*, **53**, 391–399.

Kendler, K.S., Karkowski, L.M., and Prescott, C.A. (1999). Causal relationship between stressful life events and the onset of major depression. *American Journal of Psychiatry*, **156**, 837–841.

Kendler, K.S. and Karkowski-Shuman, L. (1997). Stressful life events and genetic liability to major depression: genetic control of exposure to the environment? *Psychological Medicine*, **27**, 539–547.

Kendler, K.S., Kessler, R.C., Walters, E.E., *et al.* (1995). Stressful life events, genetic liability, and onset of an episode of major depression in women. *American Journal of Psychiatry*, **152**, 833–842.

Kendler, K.S., Neale, M.C., Kessler, R.C., *et al.* (1994). The clinical characteristics of major depression as indices of the familial risk to illness. *British Journal of Psychiatry*, **165**, 66–72.

Ketter, T.A., Andreason, P.J., George, M.S., *et al.* (1996). Anterior paralimbic mediation of procaine-induced emotional and psychosensory experiences. *Archives of General Psychiatry*, **53**, 59–69.

Kimonides, V.G., Spillantini, M.G., Sofroniew, M.V., *et al.* (1999). Dehydroepiandrosterone antagonizes the neurotoxic effects of corticosterone and translocation of stress-activated protein kinase 3 in hippocampal primary cultures. *Neuroscience*, **89**, 429–436.

Klysner, R., Bent-Hansen, J., Hansen, H.L., *et al.* (2002). Efficacy of citalopram in the prevention of recurrent depression in elderly patients: placebo-controlled study of maintenance therapy. *British Journal of Psychiatry*, **181**, 29–35.

Lesch, K.P. (2001). Serotonergic gene expression and depression: implications for developing novel antidepressants. *Journal of Affective Disorders*, **62**, 57–76.

Liotti, M., Mayberg, H.S., Brannan, S.K., *et al.* (2000). Differential limbic-cortical correlates of sadness and anxiety in healthy subjects: implications for affective disorders. *Biological Psychiatry*, **48**, 30–42.

Lotrich, F.E., Pollock, B.G., and Ferrell, R.E. (2001). Polymorphism of the serotonin transporter: implications for the use of selective serotonin reuptake inhibitors. *American Journal of Pharmacogenomics*, **1**, 153–164.

Luciana, M. and Nelson, C.A. (1998). The functional emergence of prefrontally-guided working memory systems in four- to eight-year-old children. *Neuropsychologia*, **36**, 273–293.

Lupien, S.J., de Leon, M., de Santi, S., *et al.* (1998). Cortisol levels during human aging predict hippocampal atrophy and memory deficits. *Nature Neuroscience*, **1**, 69–73.

Lupien, S.J., Nair, N.P., Briere, S., *et al.* (1999). Increased cortisol levels and impaired cognition in human aging: implication for depression and dementia in later life. *Review of Neuroscience*, **10**, 117–139.

Lynch, M. and Cicchetti, D. (1998). Trauma, mental representation, and the organization of memory for mother-referent material. *Development and Psychopathology*, **10**, 739–759.

Mayberg, H.S., Liotti, M., Brannan, S.K., *et al.* (1999). Reciprocal limbic-cortical function and negative mood: coverging PET findings in depression and normal sadness. *American Journal of Psychiatry*, **156**, 675–682.

McDonald, A.J. (1998). Cortical pathways to the mammalian amygdala. *Progress in Neurobiology*, **55**, 257–332.

McDonald, A.J., Shammah-Lagnado, S.J., Shi, C., *et al.* (1999). Cortical afferents to the extended amygdala. *Annals of the New York Academy of Sciencesi*, **877**, 309–338.

McEwen, B.S. and Sapolsky, R.M. (1995). Stress and cognitive function. *Current Opinion in Neurobiology*, **5**, 205–216.

Meyer, J.H., Kapur, S., Eisfeld, B., *et al.* (2001). The effect of paroxetine on 5-HT(2A) receptors in depression: an [(18)F]setoperone PET imaging study. *American Journal of Psychiatry*, **158**, 78–85.

Mishkin, M., Suzuki, W.A., Gadian, D.G., *et al.* (1997). Hierarchical organization of cognitive memory. *Philosophical Transactions of the Royal Society of London*, **352**, 1461–1467.

Moreno, F.A., Rowe, D.C., Kaiser, B., *et al.* (2002). Association between a serotonin transporter promoter region polymorphism and mood response during tryptophan depletion. *Molecular Psychiatry*, **7**, 213–216.

Morris, J.S., Friston, K.J., Buchel, C., *et al.* (1998). A neuromodulatory role for the human amygdala in processing emotional facial expressions. *Brain*, **121**, 47–57.

Morris, J.S., Frith, C.D., Perrett, D.I., *et al.* (1996). A differential neural response in the human amygdala to fearful and happy facial expressions. *Nature*, **383**, 812–815.

Murphy, F.C., Sahakian, B.J., and O'Carroll, R.E. (1998). Cognitive impairment in depression: psychological models and clinical issues. In D. Ebert and K.P. Ebmeier (Eds.), *New Models for Depression*. Karger, Basel, pp. 1–33.

Murray, L., Woolgar, M., and Cooper, P. (2001). Cognitive vulnerability to depression in 5 year old children of depressed mothers. *Journal of Child Psychology and Psychiatry*, **42**, 891–899.

Nelson, C.A. (1998). The nature of early memory. *Preventative Medicine*, **27**, 172–179.

Neumeister, A., Konstantinidis, A., Stastny, J., *et al.* (2002). Association Between Serotonin Transporter Gene Promoter Polymorphism (5HTTLPR) and behavioral responses to tryptophan depletion in healthy women with and without family history of depression. *Archives of General Psychiatry*, **59**, 613–620.

Newcomer, J.W., Selke, G., Melson, A.K., *et al.* (1999). Decreased memory performance in healthy humans induced by stress-level cortisol treatment. *Archives of General Psychiatry*, **56**, 527–533.

Park, R.J., Goodyer, I.M., and Teasdale, J.D. (2002). Categoric overgeneral autobiographical memory in adolescents with major depressive disorder. *Psychological Medicine*, **32**, 267–276.

Patel, R., McIntosh, L., McLaughlin, J., *et al.* (2002). Disruptive effects of glucocorticoids on glutathione peroxidase biochemistry in hippocampal cultures. *Journal of Neurochemistry*, **82**, 118–125.

Paykel, E.S. (1978). The contribution of life events to the causation of psychiatric illness. *Psychological Medicine*, **8**, 245–253.

Paykel, E.S. (2001). Continuation and maintenance therapy in depression. *British Medical Bulletin*, **57**, 145–159.

Paykel, E.S., Myers, J.K., and Dienelt, M.N. (1969). Life events and depression: a controlled inquiry. *Archives of General Psychiatry*, **32**, 327–333.

Phillips, D.I. (2001). Fetal growth and programming of the hypothalamic-pituitary-adrenal axis. *Clinical Experimental Pharmacology and Physiology*, **28**, 967–970.

Phillips, D.I., Walker, B.R., Reynolds, R.M., *et al.* (2000). Low birth weight predicts elevated plasma cortisol concentrations in adults from 3 populations. *Hypertension*, **35**, 1301–1306.

Phillips, M.L., Young, A.W., Senior, C., *et al.* (1997). A specific neural substrate for perceiving facial expressions of disgust. *Nature*, **389**, 495–498.

Plomin, R., Hill, L., Craig, I.W., *et al.* (2001). A genome-wide scan of 1842 DNA markers for allelic associations with general cognitive ability: a five-stage design using DNA pooling and extreme selected groups. *Behavior Genetics*, **31**, 497–509.

Pollak, S., Cicchetti, D., and Klorman, R. (1998). Stress, memory, and emotion: developmental considerations from the study of child maltreatment. *Development and Psychopathology*, **10**, 811–828.

Pollock, B.G., Ferrell, R.E., Mulsant, B.H., *et al.* (2000). Allelic variation in the serotonin transporter promoter affects onset of paroxetine treatment response in late-life depression. *Neuropsychopharmacology*, **23**, 587–590.

Post, R.M. (1992). Transduction of psychosocial stress into the neurobiology of recurrent affective disorder. *American Journal of Psychiatry*, **149**, 999–1010.

Rice, F., Harold, G., and Thapar, A. (2002). The genetic aetiology of childhood depression: a review. *Journal of Child Psychology and Psychiatry*, **43**, 65–79.

Roozendaal, B., Phillips, R.G., Power, A.E., *et al.* (2001). Memory retrieval impairment induced by hippocampal CA3 lesions is blocked by adrenocortical suppression. *Nature Neuroscience*, **4**, 1169–1171.

Rueter, M.A., Scaramella, L., Wallace, L.E., *et al.* (1999). First onset of depressive or anxiety disorders predicted by the longitudinal course of internalizing symptoms and parent–adolescent disagreements. *Archives of General Psychiatry*, **56**, 726–732.

Sapolsky, R.M. (2000). Glucocorticoids and hippocampal atrophy in neuropsychiatric disorders. *Archives of General Psychiatry*, **57**, 925–935.

Schulze, T.G., Muller, D.J., Krauss, H., *et al.* (2000). Association between a functional polymorphism in the monoamine oxidase A gene promoter and major depressive disorder. *American Journal of Medical Genetics*, **96**, 801–803.

Scourfield, J., Martin, N., Lewis, G., *et al.* (1999). Heritability of social cognitive skills in children and adolescents. *British Journal of Psychiatry*, **175**, 559–564.

Sheline, Y.I. (2000). 3D MRI studies of neuroanatomic changes in unipolar major depression: the role of stress and medical comorbidity. *Biological Psychiatry*, **48**, 791–800.

Silberg, J., Pickles, A., Rutter, M., *et al.* (1999). The influence of genetic factors and life stress on depression among adolescent girls. *Archives of General Psychiatry*, **56**, 225–232.

Teasdale, J.D. and Barnard, P.J. (1993). *Affect, Cognition and Change: remodelling depressive thought.* Lawrence Erlbaum Associates, Hillsdale, New Jersey.

Teasdale, J.D., Lloyd, C.A., and Hutton, J.M. (1998). Depressive thinking and dysfunctional schematic mental models. *British Journal of Clinical Psychology*, **37**, 247–257.

Vazquez, D.M. (1998). Stress and the developing limbic-hypothalamic-pituitary-adrenal axis. *Psychoneuroendocrinology*, **23**, 663–700.

Whalen, P.J., Rauch, S.L., Etcoff, N.L., *et al.* (1998). Masked presentations of emotional facial expressions modulate amygdala activity without explicit knowledge. *Journal of Neuroscience*, **18**, 411–418.

Yamamoto, M., Suhara, T., Okubo, Y., *et al.* (2002). Age-related decline of serotonin transporters in living human brain of healthy males. *Life Science*, **71**, 751–757.

Index